WHAT'S SAID IN THE CHAIR, STAYS IN THE CHAIR

(So get in my chair and I'll tell you)

Debbie McRoberts

ISBN: 1546645756
ISBN-13: 9781546645757
Library of Congress Control Number: 2017909869
CreateSpace Independent Publishing Platform, North Charleston, SC

This book is dedicated to the late John Estrada,
for bringing my stories to life.

Doing hair has always been a passion of mine. It allows me to be artistic and creative, making people look and feel their best while bonding with them, and, becoming part of their lives. I never put too much thought into it beyond that. The truth is, there is way more to doing hair than, doing hair. The relationships you build. The trust you accrue from your clients. The best feeling is having your first request appointment from a returning client who believes in you. As you walk out to greet him or her, you smile just enough to not seem overly excited, tipping the client off that he or she is the king or queen of your growing business that will form your hair empire.

You don't want clients to feel as if they are the first ones to arrive at the party, or that they are the only guests. You must conduct yourself as if you have been doing hair forever, exuding confidence in a way that you yourself believe it—as if each step you take includes cut hair particles falling off you and bowing before you as you walk out to greet them. You throw around words such as "exfoliate" or "emulsify" while engaging the client in the mirror. I used to think the mirror was my enemy, worried my immature expressions of eye rolling and unawareness of others would blow my cover. But now, I use it to my advantage. I own my game. My area is clean; I have nothing to hide. I am seasoned!

Hair stylists are insecure. We always think we are not good enough. When we get a call from a client who wants to talk to us, we assume he or she is unhappy with our services, even if he or she has followed us around for years. Getting calls from clients who loved what you did is rare. Usually they want you to fix something. It never occurred to me that I'd have to deal with hair politics. I just wanted to do hair.

Doing hair, for me, is like breathing. It just feels as though it was the right path for me, and it has been an amazing journey that I would not change. I have made many friends that are like family. I have watched kids grow up, clients get married, and clients get divorced. Seen hairlines recede, hair color fade, and hair grow. I've seen lots of hair grow…It does grow, and some people seem shocked by this, as if their color or cut should last until the end of time. It grows, believe me, or I would not have a job or material to write this book. I am happy. Let's all eat healthy, take vitamins, and grow more hair.

There is not much I have not heard or seen. Cutting hair has allowed me to buy a house and raise my kids. And for that, I am grateful. I thank each and every one of my clients for their continued support, friendship, and quirky ways, and for making me want to get up and go to this career choice of mine. The job I love.

GROWING UP SMALL

I grew up in a small town that no longer exists and feels one thousand miles away. But if I drove, I could be there in four hours, standing in the place my house once stood. I could be standing in the front yard, recognizing the two trees I used to tie a rope to and spend the afternoon jumping over, moving the rope up higher with each accomplished mark. As I look at the place now, there are trees everywhere. My kids are amazed at how I can pick the two familiar trees out of the lineup.

The road that led up to my house is overgrown with weeds and newly planted trees that have sprouted up quickly over the abandoned years. You have to climb carefully now through a barbed-wire fence to approach the place I once lived, feeling like a trespasser on the land that holds my childhood. I stand where my house once stood, remembering the place where my bedroom was and, as if looking out the window, I notice the view I had. Up on a hill was a tether ball where I would spend many days outside playing until the sun went down, when I could no longer see to hit the ball.

Up above the house is another dirt road. It was not used much, but it is the road that led to my best friend's house. The dirt roads are the roads where I learned to ride my bike, that skinned my knees when I crashed. I look at the scars now, and they bring me back to my childhood. The sweet memories that I have stored away. The ones worth getting out, dusting off, and really remembering.

I stand in the place once again where my bedroom was, picturing all it held. One night, my sister and I had a fight about who would turn the light out. It was a nightly occurrence my mother grew tired of, so she took our lightbulb away for a week. It was the wintertime then, and it got dark early. After a week in the dark, we made a chart, and every night before one of us would turn out the light, that person would put an *X* by her name so there would be no denying whose turn it was. We cut out pictures of our idols from *Teen Magazine* and taped their heads to our lampshade. The glow of Shaun Cassidy's face was enough for us not to fight about who turned the light out again.

Now, I see the living room and remember how I was obsessed with *The Gong Show*. I had to watch it every weekday at noon. I dreamed of being on the show. I just knew that they could not gong a little girl, and I would win. I often wrote the info down about how to be a contestant and gave it to my mom. She would always tell me it was filmed a long way away, and we would have to fly on a plane, and we couldn't do that. I didn't understand the big deal. No one in the family had flown before, and it was expensive. But if I were to win, I could pay my mom back, so I got ready just in case she changed her mind. I would stand on the coffee table as my stage, with the end of the jump rope as my microphone, and watch myself in the mirror that was stationed above the couch as I sang "You Light up My Life" along with Debbie Boone. "So many nights, I sit by my window, waiting for someone to come along." My brother would always come along while I was practicing, in mid-high note and tell me to shut up. Then one day, my forty-five record received an anonymous scratch, and that was the end of my childhood dream.

I had a tape recorder and would tape *Donny and Marie* and later play it back in my bedroom while wearing my purple socks. I found I could sing both parts. Turned out, I was a little bit country and a little bit rock 'n' roll. I would also tape *The Brady Bunch*. Before the show was to start, I would notify my brother that there would be a recording in progress and beg him to be quiet during my taping. He would make me so mad when he would belch or pass gas loudly and ruin my taping. I was polite when his shows were on. I actually left the room, and I wished he would pay me the same courtesy. I wasn't interested in watching *Planet of the Apes* or *Star Trek*, afraid of liking the same shows and bonding right there in our living room.

We used to fight and wreak havoc with each other. I guess since I was the baby of the family, my brother and sister used to think our parents favored me. In my eyes, they treated us all the same. But then, if that were true, there would be nothing to blame our feuding on. I grew tired of my brother sharing his gaseous moments with me, and I found a way to get even. I went to the kitchen to retrieve a ziplock bag and took it back up to my bedroom. My mom had served beans for dinner, and they had kicked in. I passed gas into the ziplock bag and sealed it up as quickly as I could. I wasn't sure it would work, but if it did, it would be one of my most brilliant ideas to date. I went into my brother's room to give him the surprise. I told him I had something special for him, and even though it didn't look like much, an invisible secret was inside, and he had to open it in his face so it wouldn't get out. I told him he would see what was in there if he followed my instructions. He did just that, and to my amusement, it worked! It was contained and awaiting to be part of my payback. I got a little bit even with him that night.

My sister and I would play *I Dream of Jeannie*. We got a pop bottle and pink and blue markers. I always got to play the role of Jeannie since I looked more like her with my blonde hair. My sister had darker hair, so the role of Jeannie's sister went to her. Besides, she sounded like her when she said, "Jeannie, darling..." Sometimes we got grounded to our room. I guess it was a crime to pick the coffee table up on one end and use it for Barbie's amusement as if she were in Disneyland, going down a big slide. Mothers frown on such things. We would be bored in our room when it wasn't our idea to be in there, so we would pretend it was the sewer, and we had been flushed down there. We stood on our headboards and dove onto our beds, pretending to be swimming around. Nothing like growing up in a small town; it forces you to use your imagination. I think that is why I am easily amused. I can find humor in the little daily happenings. I crack myself up and have been labeled a dork by others in the past, but I think it stems from having to entertain myself as a child.

We only had one bathroom that all five of us had to take turns sharing. I thought this was normal. After all, I noticed while watching the *Brady Bunch* that six kids had to share and deal with the same fight we did. The hard part was my stepdad. He spent a lot of time in there at night. If I woke in the night and had to use the bathroom, I was out of luck. It was as if he were camping and that was his tent. One night, I went to the kitchen and got a bowl out of the cupboard and took it to my closet. I thought I was dying, and there was no way I was going to go outside in the dark. The crickets out there were calming, but the coyotes terrified me. In the morning, I disposed of the bowl's contents, washed it out, and put it back in the cupboard. I told my sister about it since I didn't want her to have to use it for cereal. Whenever my mom served something in *the* bowl, we passed it along to my brother. Then we laughed as he sat there eating from it. After all, he was mean to me and would throw his Lincoln Logs down the hall and hit me in the head while I slept. Had I put some thought into it, I would not have thrown them back his way. In time, I would have enough logs to build a log cabin where Ken and Barbie could have lived happily ever after. Things were always flying down the hall at me from my brother's room. How was I so lucky to have my bed in his throwing path? One of the worst things were his smelly socks. Sometimes I would wake in the morning to find one sleeping with me on my pillow. Finally my sister shared the secret of the bowl with him, and we all passed it to the next person, each ending up with it at times. Funny it never occurred to me to throw it away.

Traveling away from town, I remember all of the bus rides to and from school. One day, my friend and I decided to hide our gum chewing since it was forbidden on the bus. My friend's aunt was the bus driver, so I thought she would be lenient with us if we got caught. We took our coats off and zipped them over our heads, making our own little cozy tents. Inside my cozy tent, I chewed to my heart's content, blowing bubbles until I heard Aunt Bernice asking if we were chewing gum. Was it that obvious? She stopped the bus and came back and unzipped our coats. We were caught! I didn't even have time to get the traces of the popped bubble off my upper lip. I would have swallowed it, but my sister told me it would stick to my insides for seven years. Aunt Bernice made us scrape gum from under the cafeteria tables for a week. There is something about chewing gum when you are not supposed to. I have learned how to tuck it away in my cheek, so tightly that it's a secret with myself.

Growing up in a small town, you have to make your own fun. My friends and I would pack a lunch and go up in the mountains for the better part of the day, making forts and pretending to be Sacajawea. We dropped breadcrumbs along the way in case we got lost. As if getting lost was ever an option; we lived in a town where everyone knew us. We had big imaginations and never ran out of things to do. The night would appear very quickly. The bats would come out and dive at us. My brother told me that if a bat were to get in my hair, it would make a nest and live there forever. That thought terrified me. I pictured this huge hive of hair about three feet high with a bat living there. Sort of like Marge Simpson, only I didn't know who she was back then. When I saw her in my adult years, it brought back memories of the "Bat hive."

Moving away from my childhood town was a devastation. It was a mill town that was government owned called Kinzua, Oregon. The mill was closing, and they were going to tear the town down, so we had to move. The concept of not having anything left was not one I could wrap my head around. I heard that it would become a ghost town and pictured ghosts living there and wondered where they would dwell if everything was gone. This would remain a mystery until I revisited the torn-down town in my later years. The roads were still there, but everything else seemed so bare. The rock pond in the backyard was still unscathed, but seemed less durable. Now, when I see it, I call it my Kinzua ruins. A friend of mine always teases me about where I came from. He calls it "that knife town, Ginsu." He knows it is Kinzua.

I wanted to move where my best friend was moving. I pleaded my case and lost. When I first saw our new town, I couldn't believe it. There were paved roads, lights on the buildings, and traffic lights. Back home, we had a couple of stop signs and a stop flap. All of the houses were brown, and then we pulled up in front of our new white house with blue trim. I couldn't believe it. We were going to live in the white house!

I missed my best friend, but soon felt better once I laid eyes on the boy next door. He was two years older and the cutest boy I had ever seen since the orange-fingered boy I was in love with from the age of four until he moved away at the end of fifth grade. His fingers were always orange from eating Cheetos. He wasn't actually my boyfriend; in truth, he acted as if he didn't like me at all. He would always run from me, but I never grew tired of chasing after him with puckered lips. I would make kissing noises as I got closer, letting him believe I wasn't afraid to kiss him. I don't know if I would have actually kissed him had I caught him, but I was always a step behind him. We rode the teeter-totter, and he got me in the air and pointed at something behind me. I fell for it every time and crashed down as he jumped off and started the chase all over again. This was when I knew he loved me. When I heard he was moving away, I could not process it. It was the worst news I had ever received in my life.

The boy next door made me so nervous. For the first time in my life, I was speechless. His feathered hair was perfect. Every strand had its place. He parted it down the middle and years later told me he used Max for Men hairspray, and when the wind would hit his hair, it would fly up, like wings. I did witness it, and it was pretty spectacular. The first day of school, he came to the bus stop looking like a million bucks. He was wearing Hash jeans. I had no idea what kind of jeans they were, the brand, but I had enough sense to know I was envious. I wanted to be "in" the way he was but knew, somehow, I had fallen short. For starters, my mom had a hard time finding pants that would fit me, since I was so small, and when she would find some, she would buy several of them; I looked as if I wore the same pair of jeans day in and day out. I used to draw on them, so the kids who sat by me in class would know they were a different pair than the day before and not think I only owned one pair.

As I got on the bus, I decided not to sit alone, but rather, I sat by a fashionable girl who looked to be about my age. I promptly introduced myself and had a feeling we would be the kind of friends who were more just acquaintances, not the secret-sharing type. She was so pretty, and I was feeling a little out of my league. I was missing my best friend, who I was certain was having similar new-school issues. Later she wrote to me about her experiences. I loved getting her letters. I would open them so fast and read them so swiftly at first and then again in a slower, taking-it-all-in kind of pace. I wrote back as soon as I could and awaited another mail call from her. We were both the peewees of our school. In all of the school pictures, we were always the two short girls on the ends, sort of like little bookends that I liked to think held the photo together. All of the girls in my new school seemed too big, so mature, so developed. Where did I fit in? Sure, I had the longest hair, and everyone told me they loved it. I was the girl with the long blonde hair, and it became my identity.

I could not wait to get home and spy on the cute boy next door after school. He rode his bike past my house and I watched him from my bedroom window, hiding behind the corner of the curtain. I never grew tired of spying on him, especially as I got older. One day, a friend and I went over to his house to play basketball. He was a big motorcycle rider. He and his friends were going to go change their clothes to go riding. Since I was the smaller one, I climbed on my friend's back to look through the bedroom window as his friends were changing. I was giving my friend the full report when one of the boys saw me while only in his underwear. I was telling her that I was spotted, but she would not let me down. Turned out, she was mad I was the one getting the view, not her. My neighbor came out with a big bowl of water and chased after me. I could only run so fast without shoes, and he poured the water over my perfectly feathered hair. I never tried that again. You just don't mess with the hair.

Going into high school, I felt so small. I was only eighty-nine pounds, and all of the other girls were developed. All of these breast exercises, and nothing seemed to work. "We must, we must, we must increase our bust...the bigger the better, the tighter the sweater, they all depend on us." I was just as shy as I was flat chested. A group of boys would hang out at a heater located near my locker. One of the boys always called me Chicken Little. He always scared me since he was an upperclassman: the loud and proud type. He loved picking on other students and getting all up in their business. He dragged me down the hall by my feet while making clucking noises. I carried all of my books for the first four classes so I could avoid chicken calls at my locker. This went on for two years, then he graduated and moved on. I saw the mean boy at a class reunion eight years later, and he asked if I was Chicken Little. I nodded my head yes, and he said I had hatched. I told him that this was a great moment. He was fat and bald. I then knew I had finally grown into myself.

The end of my sophomore year in high school, I skipped school with two other girls. We didn't want to run three miles in PE. I was having a good hair day and was all dressed up. As we were driving away from school, I saw a friend of my parents and thought it best to hide so my parents wouldn't find out I was skipping. My friend who was driving turned the corner and, when she did, the car door flew open. The cassette tape box fell out, spilling cassettes all over the road, and then I started falling out of the car in slow motion. First, my toes were dragging, then my knee hit the pavement, followed by my hip and the rest of me. My first thought was that I tore the dress I was borrowing or was getting blood on it, so I hiked it up and started chasing the car. My friend apparently didn't know I had fallen out. She kept driving up the street. This big commotion caused a stir, and the family friend came running to my aid, telling me he would call my parents. Great! Now I was caught since I had to go to the hospital to get the gravel extracted from my knee and have a tetanus shot. This was the day before cheerleading tryouts. As I woke in the morning, stiff, unable to move my arm from the shot—a bruised hip and ego—I decided to go ahead and try out for the squad, despite my pain and fear. We had to try out in front of the whole school. I limped out there, and as I saw all of the kids looking at me, I started my cheer feeling no pain. Out of the sea of fellow students, I immediately saw the boy I had a crush on, making the process more painful.

A kid yelled out, "Daredevil Debbie!" Another yelled, "Stunt woman!" I think I got the pity vote, because after all that, I was on the cheer squad.

The next time I was riding in the car with my mom and we came onto the place where I had fallen out of the moving car, she asked, "Is this where you bit the dust?" Years later I finally told her the truth about skipping school, avoiding running three miles in PE, adorned with a borrowed dress and exceptional hair. Originally, she thought it had been before school, and that we had driven to a friend's house to get her PE clothes. I am sure the truth hurt all these years later, but I was the one who had to live with the scars.

Before high school graduation, my best friend and I were moving to an apartment for the summer, before we moved away to the big city. She had been staying in a fifth-wheel trailer out in the driveway of her parents' home. I was taking a load of her things out to put in the car when I heard her say my name. As I looked back at her, I saw she had a gun, pointed in my direction. I don't know why, but I ducked. The gun went off, and I thought I had been shot. I dropped the box of her things, made it down the three steps of the fifth wheel, and fell to the ground, looking up at the blue sky. Knowing I had been shot and was going to die, I found peace in the calmness of the day. I heard her dad ask what that noise was. My friend yelled back that it was a firecracker. She came running to me, telling me to get up before her dad came over, saying that I had not been shot. I couldn't believe it. I needed help. I was going to die right there. I heard her dad drive away, feeling my chances of help were diminished. Finally, I realized it wasn't so bad; I didn't feel any pain. She urged me to get up, upset with me for lying there in the gravel. It took a moment for this to process. I was getting a second chance and was going to get to graduate after all. Good thing my instincts told me to duck, because the gun did go off. The bullet went through the wall of the fifth wheel and landed in the car door of her grandpa's Pinto, leaving gunpowder on my face. I was so upset with my friend, and she didn't see the big deal. I walked around like a zombie for two weeks thinking of what could have happened. Whenever I go to town, I visit her parents and have to go see the bullet. One time, the car was gone. I asked the dad what happened to the car, and he said he sold it. I asked if he'd ever noticed the bullet in the door, and he said he had; he thought it was a stray bullet. Really? Are there stray bullets flying around? I had never been aware of them before. Now, I'd be on the lookout. I told him how it had gotten there, about the day he'd asked about the noise and had driven away. He said he was going to tell his daughter that he traced the bullet from the Pinto car door and ask how it came from his gun to see if she'd come clean.

It is always fun to go visit my mom and confess things to her that I did as a child. I can barely get the story out since I am laughing so hard, and she is sitting there with that look on her face that sends me into hysterics. I used to put pieces of my meat in these holes under the table. It seemed we always had meat and potatoes for dinner, and I would be the last one sitting there, staring at the unfinished meal. I chewed a piece of meat, and it just grew in my mouth, doubling in size, making it impossible to swallow. And what were those stringy things? I had rather large tonsils, and it didn't seem to matter the size of the bite; I just could not get it down.

One night, I packed all of my meat in my cheek and said, as politely as I could, "Excuse me. I have to go to the bathroom." When I was out of my mother's sight, I saw my sister looking at me. I pointed to my cheek and pointed at her while laughing. I thought it was funny that she hadn't been as clever as I had been and that she had to remain at the table and finish her meal. I could have flushed the fleshy bite, but my sister had been mean to me, so I spit it under her mattress. We had bunk beds at the time that had fallen. She was climbing up to the top bunk one night and, luckily, I was not in bed yet. It collapsed, so her mattress was on the floor while the bed was being repaired. A month later, when the bed was finally fixed, my mom found the meat under the mattress. I acted as though I didn't know what the green wad was. Later in my confession, she found the truth.

HOW IT ALL BEGAN

Growing up in a small town, we didn't have hairdressers. Back then, the job title was beauty operator. Whenever someone calls me that, I have to stop and say, "Stand back everybody. I'm operating beauty in here."

Since there was no beauty operator, my mom decided to set up her own kitchen salon and attempt to "trim" my hair. My hair was very long, as in the sometimes-I-sit-on-it length. I pretended to be like Cher, and I gave it that toss away, tossing it sassily behind my back, with my elbow glued to my hip and my hand stretched out forward like a drooping flower demanding to be kissed. I used to float in the bathtub and pretend I was a mermaid. I would move my head back and forth and let my hair dance in the water. I loved my long locks. They were healthy and shiny, as my grandma would say. I acted like a movie star and brushed my hair while counting. I did one hundred strokes, like Marsha Brady. This act only lasted maybe three nights, tops, but there was no denying it. My hair rocked.

When I was in the seventh grade, I decided to get bangs. I had moved to a bigger town where there was a salon just up the street, forcing my mom to close down her kitchen cuts. Now I was to go to the mother of a boy in my reading class. The night before, I hardly slept. I don't know how many times I tried to picture what they would look like by holding a big strand of my own hair across my forehead to form the illusion of bangs. All day, I watched the clock and, to my excitement, it was time for my appointment. They were cut in a matter of minutes, and I was thrilled with them. So thrilled that I left the salon, ran all the way home, and forgot to pay for my service. The next day, I ended up giving the boy in my reading class the money to give to his mom.

As time went on, I toyed with the idea of having more of a feathered look. Farrah was hot at the time, and if I couldn't have her eraser tip nipples, then I would at least have her hair. My step grandma would cut my stepdad's hair in her kitchen, so I called to ask her about cutting my hair, and she invited me over. My hair was still to my waist, but we just cut the sides to make it feather back. I went home to play with it and decided I wanted the length shorter. She had me come back over, and she cut the length up to my shoulders. I was so nervous. I couldn't tell what she was doing, and then it occurred to me that my stepdad always wore a hat. Was that a sign? I guess when someone offers to cut your hair, you assume he or she knows what he or she is doing, no questions asked. So I just sat in the chair in the middle of the kitchen and focused on the leftovers since there was no mirror in sight. I remember thinking, "At least give me a shiny toaster, something where I can get an idea of what is going on." When it was finished, I went to the bathroom to check it in the mirror. But what if I didn't like it? What could I say? I didn't pay her. She was doing me a favor. I'd better like it. What if it went awry and I hated what she did to my hair? She was family. I would have to sit there with her, sharing a Thanksgiving dinner. I imagined I would help clear the table when the meal was finally over and, stepping into the familiar kitchen, learn that she did have a toaster after all.

I actually loved my shorter hair and thought my step grandma did a great job. I felt so free after all of those years with hair down my back. Then, about the third day, I woke in a panic, felt for my hair, but it was gone. I grieved for my long locks. I could no longer toss it behind my back like Cher, and there would be no more mermaid moments.

I was the curling-iron queen. I took my curling iron to school and would do a touch-up after PE. I have always been obsessed with my hair, wanting it to look good because we all know that nothing is worse than having a bad hair day. It is true. You could be wearing a fabulous outfit, but if your hair was not right, something in the universe was just off. It is one thing to have bad hair and be in a cubical all to yourself; but when you work in a salon, everyone expects your hair to be the best.

After a year of the shorter hair, I decided to get a perm. This was a disaster in itself. My hair was big and puffy, and there was nothing that was going to tame it. Not even my beloved curling iron. My Sunbeam three-quarter inch with steam. It was hopeless. I got it during the holiday break too, so I had to go back to school with everyone knowing what I got for Christmas. I was excited at the time and thought it to be a good idea. Knowing what I know now, as a stylist, I have to ask: Why didn't the stylist who performed that hideous permanent wave on me tell me it was a bad idea? My hair was actually bigger than me! No more healthy shine. Just dull, frizzled hair that even Farrah herself would claim unfashionable. We all know it takes time for a bad perm to grow out. It is not magically going to get healthier when it is fried in that manner. The only thing that will make it better is a conditioner called stainless steel conditioner. That is when you actually use your shears and cut it off. I went to the movies the night of the big perm. I was thankful for the darkness. I was self-conscious enough to slink down in my chair, not wanting to block anyone's view. Thank goodness the spring came and my hair healed. It feels like forever when you are waiting for a miracle. That was not the end of my perms, though. I endured it over and over. The worst was yet to come.

Five years into my career, I was working in a salon in downtown Portland where I was the only blonde stylist. My boss was on a power trip and wanted me to color my hair a dark shade. I have been a blonde my entire life. I know I would have an identity crisis if I looked into the mirror and was no longer a blonde. Not to mention, who has time to take a number and wait at the DMV to get a new driver's license photo? I have tried different colored wigs on for fun, and most other shades are not me. My boss was always showing me pictures of shorter, darker hairstyles. I finally gave in and decided to go with a shorter hairdo. I showed her the picture of what I wanted, and she agreed it would be fabulous. She would say any and every hairstyle was fabulous, even if it wasn't what the client wanted, and he or she was unhappy. She claimed that the client didn't know what he or she wanted, and that it was our job to let the client know what he or she should have. I could see if a client had no vision and needed help with what would look best for his or her hair type and facial features, but I was not going to argue with a client over what he or she should have if the client was not going to like it.

She would make me stand there at her station while she would cut and pretend to agree it was fabulous even if my taste or common sense told me otherwise. I had to keep my composure with a poker face and bluff the client that I too was in love with her hairdo, and then wait for her at the counter and take her money. It seemed I was put into the role of the salon Cinderella since I did all of the dirty work. I washed a lot of hair, rinsed perms, cleaned up after everyone, and would also wear the hat of the receptionist. I never got a dime for all of that extra work, and my hands were breaking out since they never had time to dry out. What was my title? I was only six years into my profession, but she made me feel as though I were just out of school. I was made to feel as if I didn't know a thing about cutting hair, yet my hair license was a reminder to me that I had worth. I let this salon boss beat me down until I was one of her clones, and it didn't sit well with something inside.

I was now in my boss's chair and showed her the picture of the style I wanted. She cut my hair in five minutes; I thought to make sure I wouldn't change my mind. I felt as if I were in a Jackie Chan movie, the way she was moving all around my head. I had never seen anyone cut like that—so fast. She picked up random chunks of hair and chopped them off. After she dried it, we decided to highlight it, to give it some brightness. My hair was in shock, along with the rest of me, and it would not do a thing and had no style. It was nothing like the picture. She then talked me into a five-minute perm. A five-minute perm means that you leave the perm solution on for five minutes, enough to change the texture of the hair. I think she forgot about me, or set me aside while she was chopping another client's hair, because what felt like an hour later, when she took the perm rods out—that moment of truth—my hair had melted. When I grabbed and pulled on it, it actually stretched.

I went home early that day to do some crying and, wouldn't you know it, that night, right there on ABC, was the Miss USA Pageant. There were all of those beauties strutting their stuff with all of their long, shiny hair. It was like hair candy, taunting me with the reality that I was in an ugly short hair nightmare. The next day when I awoke and realized I really did look like a Q-tip, I felt like I wanted revenge.

Staring in the mirror, I saw that it looked as if I had been to the fair and had cotton candy on my head. The thought of calling in sick crossed my mind; in fact, hibernating until my hair was better sounded like a good plan, but I decided to go to work and return to the scene of the crime.

When I went to work, clients asked me what happened to my beautiful long hair. I told them to ask my boss. She did not like this attention. After she knew my hair was a disaster and actually admitted it was, she used me as a learning experience. We all sat around my fuzz head and talked about how we would make sure to listen to clients' needs when they came in and wanted a change— and not to promise the picture.

In my mind, my revenge left me wondering if I should offer to cut her hair and leave it an undesirable mess, that would send her home to cry. But I couldn't do that. She was my boss, and it would be bad advertisement. My mind was entertained with such scenarios, but I was too nice to follow through and eventually found new employment.

I promised a picture only one time. An older lady was in my chair, showing me a picture of a younger lady's style. Knowing her hair was a lot thinner than that of the gal in the photo, I started cutting without pulling out my insurance. The insurance we use when we tell them it will not be exactly like the picture, due to hair texture, the amount of hair; a cowlick perhaps. The lady made a comment to me that it looked nothing like the lady's hair in the picture. I really thought she knew her hair was nothing like the lady's hair in the photo. She seemingly only had three hairs on her head. I mean, come on, anyone could see that. This was when I learned my lesson that you never promise the picture. But when it did turn out to resemble the picture, you were a hair God. I used to get all of these high school girls in for their prom hairdos. A girl would bring an unrealistic picture, and I would tell her that we would work together, and if at any moment I placed a bobby pin she didn't like, she could tell me right away. Otherwise, hold your peace.

Some of them would get snotty and tell me, "It doesn't look like Cindy Crawford." I so wanted to say in return, "Well, honey, you don't look like Cindy Crawford, either!" But I didn't want to ruin their big night, and I learned to bite my tongue.

After the melting hair experience and the boss from hell, I decided to move to a different salon where I rented my station and could be more of the boss of me. It was time to get away from the negative comments she made, such as telling me I looked like a Safeway checker. I went to Safeway one night to check out the checkers, and it turned out it was not a compliment. Some of them wore aprons, which could resemble the aprons hair stylists used to keep hair and color off their clothes, but they also wore uniforms. My boss obviously hated my clothes and took it upon herself to shop for me, taking the cost out of my paycheck. Then she told me I had to wear the clothes she picked out for me to work since I was "on stage," and I could wear whatever I wanted at home. I didn't want to be on her stage. I was tired of rehearsing my lines, tired of being the type of actor she wanted me to be. It was time to find a new venue where I could really shine and be the top billing actress on my own stage, my own leading lady.

The last perm I had, my hair didn't melt or stretch, but it had that smell that made anyone who got within six feet from me wonder where the smell was coming from. It smelled like a wet dog. Not the kind that had gone to the dog wash place and had been scrubbed with oatmeal shampoo, but the kind that had been out in the rain after rolling around in a chicken coop. I decided to give up perms. I had gone white water rafting the day after the smelly perm, and for all of us who have had perms know, you cannot wash it for forty-eight hours, or it will weaken the curl. Now, why didn't the stylist who gave me my first perm share this bit of knowledge with me? I would have been up sudsing all night! During this rafting trip, I went down a twenty-foot waterfall, fell in the rapids, and had wet hair all the way home, smelling up the van. It was embarrassing when everyone had that look on their faces of smelling something bad. Looking at the pinched faces of my fellow passengers made me want to give it all up.

I have clients who will be on my schedule for a perm. I will call them and ask them what they are doing. Why are they scheduled for a perm? They will tell me they want a change, and I will ask them if they are just going to wash and wear it. If they are, and they are under seventy, then they are too young for the wash and wear. I tell them to ask me again when they are that age. I really try to avoid the perm unless I know the person will benefit from it. I have actually told a client, and I did say these words, "I hate to say this...oh great, here goes...you need a perm." I would never have offered it up unless I knew for sure it would change her life, making her hair easier for her while looking good. I permed her hair right there on the spot. She called her husband first, not to ask his permission, but to tell him to take the chicken out of the freezer; she would be home later. She was getting a perm. His response was not what I would have thought. He said, "Now don't be starting that." "Starting what?" I asked. We were not opening up a can of worms here. I knew what I was doing and finally gave the go ahead. I told her from now on not to share perm time with him. Besides, most men don't even know when their wives have been in to get their hair done. They could have a drastic change and it could go unnoticed for weeks. I called one of my guy clients to tell him to notice his wife's hair, that I had given her a new hairdo and it would mean a lot to her to know he was paying attention, letting him score some points.

In high school, after studying the stylist who cut my hair, I decided I could cut my hair myself. Clients actually think this. They watch, take notes, and think it looks easy. The bilevel was popular at the time, so I went for it. In my bathroom with what I believe were the kitchen scissors—the ones my mom used to cut the heads off the trout that we had caught the summer of '75 (Don't try this at home)—and went for it. I transformed myself into a female Billy Ray Cyrus, and I thought I was looking good. Now I could really feather my hair back on the sides and still have some length in the back. I believe it was called a Kentucky Waterfall, where it was all business in the front and a party going on in the back. Now when a client uses the term "feather," I try not to cringe, thinking it's old school.

After my own barbering, if you will, my friends asked me who cut my hair. I smiled and told them it was me. They wanted me to cut their hair. I couldn't believe it. After one self-cut, I already had their trust? My family was making a trip to the big city of Bend, Oregon, so I was on the lookout for a pair of haircutting scissors. I didn't know the technical term for "scissors" was "shears." I went to K-Mart and found a pair for twelve dollars. I thought that was a lot to invest since I wasn't going to charge for my work. Could I call it that? Work? What if they didn't like it? I used to cut my boyfriend's hair out in his front yard. He would go in and inspect it right after, while I would wait and worry for his reaction, with total relief that there wasn't a toaster nearby for him to watch me in, thankful for the blind cut. He asked me to cut more off around the ears. I wasn't sure how to just cut more off around the ears, but I had my game face on and made my way through it.

There were so many curling iron traumas. You had to take caution. If you got the hot barrel too close to your scalp, or hairline, it would really burn and leave a mark. It was a touchy subject if the burn was on your neck. A few days into the healing process, it dries up and starts looking like a hickey. One time, after a curling iron burn on my neck that was in the hickey faze, I ran into a man I used to date. I tried to hide my neck, worried he would think it was a hickey. I pointed it out and told him it was an actual burn. He just looked at me and walked away as if he didn't believe me. Who would make something up like that? I am a professional hair stylist, and I burn my neck! One time in high school, as I was curling my bangs, the curling iron slipped out of my hair and landed on my nose, leaving a big red welt that later turned into a huge blister. I was in typing class at the time and had a crush on the boy who sat at my table. He kept asking me what was on the tip of my nose. I couldn't face him for the longest time, since it takes forever to heal when it's on your nose, so visible. You know everyone is looking at it. Another time, as I was rushing to curl my hair, I dropped the hot wand on my bare leg. It left the deepest burn and left me to practice some safety measures while curling my hair: never wear shorts!

I was a good detective. I solved the problem of the wanger. If you used a curling iron to feather your hair, this could happen sometimes: the wanger. One side would just "wang" out. It was so embarrassing. I would walk around holding my hair down on that side, but the moment I let go, *wang!* I even tried to lie on that side to try to calm it, but who has that kind of time in the morning? I realized that the good side—the side that didn't wang out—was my right side, and I would hold the curling iron handle downward to curl that side, but since I was right handed, when it came to the left side, I would still use my right hand to turn the curling iron handle upward, causing the wanger. I tried to use my left hand and hold it the same way as I held it on the right side, and it lay in unison with the right side. No more holding down wangers. I knew then that I was born to do hair.

MOVING TO THE BIG CITY

The summer after graduating high school, I was preparing to move to the big city, Portland, Oregon, leaving small-town life behind. I was frightened, yet so excited for all of the possibilities also moving along with me. I had only known small-town living my entire eighteen years. There were so many doors just waiting to be open, starting with the one that led me out of town, to my new adult journey. A journey that would either make me grow, or be the death of me. I was so thrilled to finally be the boss of me. No more grounding or being denied the things you were denied while living under your parents' roof, such as eating ice cream out of the carton while sitting in a certain chair labeled "Dad." These are the normal thoughts of a teenage mind. However, teenagers can only act upon them if they aren't in need of support and funding from the parental units. It is a self-sufficient awareness that can only happen if they are, self-sufficient.

My mom didn't want me to leave. She sat up in my room crying, asking me not to go—to stay and continue working at the A&W where I was making about $3.75 an hour. Although, it was cool, and I was the carhop. I wore the money belt as if it had all the power. There was nothing like the feeling of carrying a tray of food, hooking it onto the diner's car window with the sound of the money belt banging against my brown polyester pants, which they made me wear, as I walked. It was the sweetest sound of power, and I knew how to use it. I could make change so fast; the fries never had time to cool. But I was ready for something more. Something bigger than me. The big city was calling my name.

My mom told me bad things would happen in the city. I was led to believe I would be shot just for walking out in the open or kidnapped if I were alone. After all, we would watch the Portland news, and it did cover all of these cases. There were always shootings, robberies, and kidnappings. Now I was afraid more than ever! I had to be aware of my surroundings at all times. It put a fear in me. I was going to be out in the big world, no longer in my small-town bubble, unable to trust strangers. I had to be on guard at all times.

I moved to Portland with the friend who almost shot me, since I was a forgiving sole. I was following her in my car, and her parents were our guides ahead of her. As we neared the big city, I really felt awake. We stopped at our first red light, and I was so afraid I would be left behind if I didn't tail them. I dared to look around and saw a bench. It had the words "Rent a Bench" on it. I couldn't believe it. You actually had to rent a bench to sit down in the city? Was it free on Sundays? How much was it? Was it based on the honor system? Was there a coin drop box somewhere, and what if you didn't have change? I saw a couple of people sitting on the bench. It looked as if they were getting their money's worth on account of my first big city public display of affection. I thought I would just sit on the sidewalk next to it to mock it, if I dared to sit out in the open. Back home, all of the benches were free.

I mentioned this bench fee to my friend's dad as we arrived at our new apartment. I wondered why anyone would want to sit in the same spot. If I rented a bench, it would be in a location closer to where I lived, so I wouldn't have to drive so far to sit on it. He just shook his head and smiled, not telling me the truth behind the benches. I really thought, for the first two years of living in the city, that you had to rent a bench to sit down. Every time something bad would happen, I would always mention how you had to rent a bench to sit down in the city. One day, a friend of mine asked me why I always mention the bench rental fee. That is when I finally found out the truth: you could rent a bench for advertisement. I had a lot to learn. Whenever I went back to my hometown, I visited my friend's parents. I told her dad that I knew now about the bench fees and that it was for advertisement, as if letting him in on this newly found knowledge. He said, "I know. I didn't want to tell you because I thought it was so cute. So innocent," he said, smirking.

I was so excited to take it all in: the city life. My friend and I used to take turns driving downtown so the other one could really look. I remember trying to see the tops of the buildings as I would put my head out the window. Back home, our tallest building was three stories. It was the post office. We used to sneak in and try to ride the elevator, but I had never been so brave. Now that I'd been in the city, I had planned to ride a lot of elevators. We used to drive around and get so lost. That is what is fun about being young. You have so much more time for exploring. More time to just go out for the day, do cartwheels until you are dizzy, drive until you are lost.

Sometimes, when I would go to the grocery store, I thought a man was following me and would probably kidnap me like my mom had talked about. I was paranoid. I would do little tests, such as going down the aisle to get peanut butter and watching to see if he was following me. If he was, then I would go to a random aisle to check again. One day, I thought this guy was really following me, so I asked the checker, "Do you see the man in the red shirt?"

"Yes," she said, and then I told her of my suspicions: that he was following me around the store. Unless we had the same shopping list, then this man was a stalker. The checker was so kind as to watch me leave and keep an eye on the man in the red shirt.

One late night while I was grocery shopping, I noticed a man who always seemed to be looking for the same items I was looking for; yet, he was empty handed and did not have a shopping cart. He made me feel as though he was following me, so I did a little test to check his shopping list and found it odd that he never took anything off the shelves. I went up to checkout, and he walked by me and left the store while giving me the horse eye. You know the look: When you look a little sideways at a person, trying to make it less obvious you are looking, trying to be inconspicuous, while still viewing. There was another fellow who left the store right after him who also gave me that look, delivering it with an eerie feeling. I told the checker about the goings on in the store, and she had the store manager walk me to my car. But then, you never know, even a security guard could be the bad guy. He could have hit the real guard over the head and then changed into his uniform. Maybe my mom just wanted me to be aware of my surroundings, but I was a wreck!

In the small town I was from, you didn't have to worry about such things. Maybe I had an active imagination or watched too much TV, but I would think people were following me behind my car. I would go around extra corners, take the long way home, and if they were still behind me, I would do one more loop just to make sure. When I finally reached my apartment, I ran up the stairs so quickly I could barely get my key in the door. Once inside, I searched. I checked all of the closets, under the bed to see if someone had made his or her way into my home. What if I'd discovered someone during these investigations? Then what? I'd say, "I just knew you would be here," and act hospitable. Throw in a "Would you fancy some tea and cookies?" I always had the phone in my hand and was ready to call for help.

Growing up and sharing a room with my sister was an interesting time. She would wake me in the middle of the night to tell me a ghost was by my bed. She would describe the old hag and what she was wearing. I would be so terrified and beg to sleep with her. I would then spend a sleepless night hiding under the covers. I had no idea why she did this. Was it for my reaction, the pure joy of making your own fun, or was our house really haunted? I did go stay a night with her in our adult years, and the same thing happened. She told me of the ghost in her house and how it did things, moved things around. She even named him Cecil. Then I remembered she once had a cactus named Cecil, so I wasn't a big believer in her ghost. That night as I lay sleeping, the bedroom door swung open with such force that it hit the wall. I could see out in the hall, but there was no one there. I got up to look around, but everyone was in bed. It freaked me out so much I ended up only staying one night. A few years later, I learned that their house was built on an old graveyard, and the mere mention of Cecil never came up again and my visits waned.

Once, a lady knocked on my door, and when I opened it, she revealed herself as a solicitor. Well, she didn't actually say that was who she was. She introduced herself and asked my name. After I told her, I decided I better not share anything else. She was from the Church of Scientology and wanted to sell me one of the Bibles. I told her I was not interested, and as I went to close the door, my phone started ringing. I closed the door, but didn't lock it since I was racing to the phone. I was talking to my dad when I turned and saw the woman standing in my entryway. She actually opened the door and came in. My dad was hard of hearing, and I was trying to explain to him that I had to go since a strange woman just came into my house. I had to think fast and couldn't believe she just opened the door and walked in after I denied her a sale.

I was in the process of making spaghetti, so I grabbed my big knife and started chopping the onion. I told her to come into the kitchen to talk to me. I was trying to play it cool, but also let her know I had a big knife. She told me she had a used Bible in her car that she could sell to me for half price. I agreed to buy it, just so I could get her out of my home.

I don't know why I was so polite in the first place and why I didn't want to offend her. After a while, through life's lessons, we realize that we are just as important as everyone else. Why do we give others more compassion than we give ourselves? All I knew that night was that I was amazed at how aggressive the people in the city were. I got mail for years from the Church of Scientology, and they had my name as "Delokee." Then one day, I noticed the mail stopped. I changed back to my maiden name twenty-two years later, and I got a phone call one night with the caller asking for Delokee. I hung up and wondered how they found me. I never had that cell phone number back then.

I guess the reason I was so scared and paranoid was from my sister and her ability to embellish in her paranormal activity beliefs, convincing me to be a believer as well. I don't know how many ghosts must have visited our bedroom in the course of a childhood, but they were all around us, in her defense. Anytime there was ever a noise that was unidentifiable, it had to be the makings of a ghost.

We were gullible kids, believing everything we heard on TV. Once, we were watching a show where this man was bit by a stray animal. He later developed rabies. We watched in horror. Weeks later, we went to the dump to dig around for treasures. There was a stray cat that my brother tried to pet, and it ended up biting him, making him think he had rabies. He told us to hurry back to the babysitter's house, for fear that he would turn into a madman and bite us too, and then we would also have rabies. He was on his bike, and we were walking, so he wanted to give us a head start. All the way to the sitter's we were way ahead of him while keeping track of his sanity.

We asked, "Are you OK?"

And he replied, "Yes." And then he told my sister that she could have his room and all of his belongings.

I remember standing there with my hands on my hips, saying, "You give her everything!" He did. He and my sister were adopted; they were biologically brother and sister. My parents didn't think they could have children, so they adopted my sister when she was three and my brother was three months. I came along two years later. My siblings were always telling me that Mom and Dad loved me more, as if they had this secret pact, only it was not a secret. I was very aware that, on my brother's death bed, he was giving my sister, not me, everything. Not that I would want anything. I just got tired of being left out, as if I would never be an option. Luckily, we made it to the babysitter's house, and he followed, no foaming of the mouth or peddling of his bike like a madman to bite and infect us. He lived, and my sister remained in my room, pointing out ghosts, weekly, at the bottom of my bed.

I am not so paranoid these days. I can go to the store and not think I am being tailed. I am actually quite comfortable, since I have been here thirty-two years. I am amazed at how small the city seems. I run into people I know all the time. I used to make a big deal out of it. If I drove and saw someone I knew, I honked at him or her; doing it up big just to get the wave back. In the little town I was from, we used to drag Main Street for hours until our curfew. It didn't take long since it wasn't that far from one end of the town to the other, and we used to wave at everyone every time we drove by. Once I went to put the visor down, and this kid, kind of the nerdy type, thought I was waving to him. He thought I liked him, and I just had the sun in my eyes. That night, the visor wave was born. I would make it a point to let one of the boys I liked know I was not waving to him. I was only putting my visor down. This ended up being our wave to each other the rest of the time I lived there.

Moving to the big city had so much to offer. There were so many strange people to look at, one had to be careful to not crash while driving. I once went to a place I didn't know was valet parking. I had no idea what this kind of parking was. As I went into the parking lot, the cars looked all aligned to me, so I pulled in and parked. I was then told I was supposed to get out and let someone park my car. What? And give someone my keys—access to my car? What kind of place was this? And on the way out, I had to tip the guy? Another thing to write home about.

I went out of town with my boyfriend to Seattle, Washington, and we were going out to dinner to a nice restaurant, and when he pulled up to the front, a guy came out of nowhere and tried to open my door. I screamed and told my boyfriend to hurry and drive away; someone was trying to get in and get me. It turned out to be, once again, valet parking. I was so embarrassed. In my defense, I never grew up with any of these amenities.

I frequented a few concerts during beauty school. It was so exciting that all my favorites were touring, and I was living in the city they wanted to visit. I bought a ticket to see Sammy Hagar. I was not on the floor level but on the next level just up from the stage. Sammy came out onto this plank, about twenty feet from me. The lights grew dim, a spotlight appeared, and he was singing to me! I looked around at everyone else, then back to him, and he was looking at me. It felt surreal, as if his fame would rub off onto me. Then he did a jump that ripped the seat of his pants, and that was my Sammy Hagar moment. As I recap the night, it dawns on me that he was probably looking at my hair. It looked just like his, only more tamed, and less sweaty. It was the '80s, and we were both rocking a perm.

29

BEAUTY SCHOOL DAYS

The first day of beauty school left me reeling with excitement. I was the first one at the school, taking my seat at the front of the class, and I was ready for the learning to begin. The second girl to arrive asked if she could sit by me. I was happy to see she was normal. As the class filed in one by one, I could pick out the ones who frightened me just a little. They were the ones who looked a little hard around the edges. I was thinking, *I'm Debbie. I drink milk. How am I going to fit in?*

Whenever we had to have a partner, I had the girl who had chosen the seat by me the first day. We became fast friends. She was from a small town as well, and she seemed to have my values. There was a rather large gal in the class who was also very loud, who would yell my name across the room that she wanted to be my partner. A couple of times I decided to be her partner, only later I was reminded of why I needed to decline in the future. Once while shampooing my hair, she held a handful of suds above my head as if she were going to drop them in my face while laughing a wicked laugh. Also, she would turn the water to freezing cold and just cackle while I tried to get away. No wonder she was always in need of a partner. She was also the one who was always in a race to be the first to finish with a task. The instructor would come over and check her work, and it was always off. She was scissor happy and cut too much. We had to use the same mannequin for the six weeks cutting class, so around the middle part of the class, she didn't have enough hair to do certain cuts or styles. She was ready for the clipper class way ahead of everyone else. I have often wondered if she was still in the hair field and if she outgrew beating the clock and dangling suds above the clients' faces, shockingly using cold water to rinse while chortling.

Every Thursday, we got to have hair mornings. It was the only time we could do one another's hair. We decided the bigger gal needed her eyebrows waxed since she was sporting the biggest unibrow I had ever seen. The kind you would write home about. I always found myself looking at it when I would talk to her. I told myself to look away, but it always grabbed my full attention. So we decided to tame the beast, and the first one in that day had the job of making sure the wax was hot and ready. There were four of us in the little room that day. Two to hold her hands, one (me) to do the waxing, and the fourth was there for support, I guess, or to just witness a monumental event. As I put the wax around the first eyebrow and lay the gauze over the wax, she already started to get nervous and made little "oohs and ouches." As I got a hold of the gauze to rip it off, I told her on the count of three I would pull. As I counted to two, I pulled, and she kicked me so hard it knocked me over, making me hit my head on the wall behind me. We were all laughing so hard, I had to run out to the bathroom in fear I would wet my pants. I got out of the room in time, as the instructor came running to see what was going on. Everyone in the room got in trouble and had to leave the room, postponing our waxing quest. No one told on me for being in there as well, and the girl had to wait another week to have the rest of the waxing completed.

As I analyzed my work in progress, I realized I should have started in the middle to part the brows; giving them their own identity. I left her looking more like a lopsided unibrow. Eyebrows should not take on the appearance of conjoined twins. When the following Thursday arrived, I was elected to finish the job. Once again, I came in early to heat the wax and could only have one other person in with us. It took a while, but we finally got the job done.

After six short weeks, when your mannequin is bald, you get to work on real people out on the floor with the advanced students. You get whatever station is available, set up shop, and await your first victim. I felt equally nervous and excited. I ended up with all the older lady roller sets. They just loved the way I back combed out their hair, and they kept my schedule busy week to week. The older ladies demanded their weekly spot, the same day and time every week. I had one lady who became very special to me. She would always snort out loud as she would laugh, so I did my best comedic act to keep her laughing. I always loved Wednesdays at one o'clock in the afternoon. I called it the laughing hour.

Since I was supporting myself through beauty school, I had to get a job to pay the rent. I would go to school from eight thirty in the morning to five o'clock at night, change out of my smock into my uniform, and head to Wendy's from five thirty to ten o'clock at night, where I was the order taker, asking, "Do you want this on a multigrain bun?" I had more fun working the register, where I got to reveal dinner orders into the microphone, but I wasn't a fan of the hat, or rather, having to tuck my bangs into my hat. I felt like a peeled onion. I have always felt more secure with a fringe around my face, and I dislike wearing things that mess with my hair.

On a slow night at Wendy's, I was told to wash the ceiling. I had no idea where to start. There was so much grease up there; once you started, you had to do the whole thing, and my shift was about over. I went to the center, where there was less traffic and hot grills coating me with hamburger fumes, and washed my name in the ceiling. DEBBIE. That was all I had time for, and after that, I had a couple of days off. As I returned to work, it was still there, and I was told when it slowed down that I had to finish the job. People going through the drive-through were at the right angle where they could see my name and would ask who Debbie was. The window cashier asked me to come to the window so I could wave. A few more days past, and I still hadn't had time to get to it. A week later, with a few days off, the manager found someone else to wash the ceiling. After eight months of fast food, I decided to get a different job at the mall selling clothes. It was a much better job, and I didn't go home smelling like burgers and fries.

While we were studying facials and skin care in school, we got to have a day where we did fantasy makeup. Once again, we had to partner up. I had my regular partner, but the large gal yelled my name across the room to call dibs on me. I didn't know how to get out of it. She was the odd man out, and I felt sorry for her, although it was her own fault for being an unpredictable partner. We let her join our group. After we finished doing makeup on one another, I came up with an idea. We just started drawing arrows on her face with purple eyeliner. One arrow led to another, and they all intersected, looking a bit busy and futuristic. The other girls said she looked like a totem pole, which made her uncomfortable, and that was the last time she ever yelled across the room again for me to be her partner.

Moving onto the nail class the first day, we received our rubber hands so we could practice putting acrylic nails on the hand. All I could do was dream of the night I was going to have with it. I could not wait to get home and put the hand in my roommate's bed. I figured if I put it toward the bottom of the bed by the wall, she would think someone was under her bed, as she would feel something and reach down to feel fingers, and then a creepy hand in her bed. I could barely contain my giddiness that night, and she thought I was being strange. I just told her I was in a good mood and had a fun day in class. I decided to go to bed early, hoping she would follow suit. I lay in my bed for what seemed like hours awaiting the showdown. Finally, I heard her in the bathroom brushing her teeth. Then into her bedroom, and then it came...the scream! She came running into my room screaming, but she found me in hysterics. I could not control it, and it gave me away that I had something to do with it. She went back into her room and threw back her covers, revealing my hand. My name was even written on the wrist. She began beating me with it, admitting she about had a heart attack. That was when I knew I was going to have fun in nail class.

We had to practice putting artificial nails on one another. They always looked good for a day. After that, they would always pop off while doing little household tasks or trying to button a blouse. They were just too long and in the way. I went out one night and needed to use the bathroom. It took me forever just to unbutton my pants. Before that, as I was closing the bathroom stall door, a nail popped off and sailed over only to land on the floor of another stall. I wanted to ask if they would pass it back to me, slide it, whatever—I just wanted it back so I could nail glue it in place. That was another thing. You had to travel with your nail glue in case of such instances. There was nothing worse than losing a nail, other than what was remaining. Nothing like four extra-long, bucket-shaped nails painted bright red next to a short stubby plain one. It always felt so naked, carrying all of that shame exposed for everyone to see, and I just knew everyone was looking at it, and all of a sudden so much disgrace existed right there in that naked nail. I just wanted to get home, repair it with the kit I took home from school in case I did lose a nail on a night out.

One night, while wearing my fake beauty school nails, I was at work manning the salad bar at Wendy's. I had to go into the walk-in refrigerator to get the items I needed and noticed we were running low on lettuce. We kept the lettuce all cut up and ready to go in a garbage can full of water. Just to clarify, I believe it was a new garbage can, solely for the purpose of storing lettuce, and it had never been used for any other purpose. As I was collecting the lettuce, I suddenly noticed I was missing a thumbnail. I had this terrible feeling it had come off and had been floating among the garbage can of lettuce. I had to find it. I kept picturing a big, bright, fake nail in someone's salad. That would be means for firing, and I needed my job, so I searched frantically, keeping this news to myself. Letting it out would only cause an upset. I sifted through, practically piece by piece, until I finally found it. I was so relieved. I could only imagine a patron picking it up with a pair of salad tongs and reporting it to my manager.

One morning, while cleaning tables at the same restaurant, I saw two men sitting, having breakfast. One read the paper, the other sat there eating, looking a little neglected since the other guy had the paper out in its full extension as if putting a shield between the two of them. Then I saw the scrambled egg on the paperless guy's forehead. My first response was to sing, "You've got egg on your face, you're a big disgrace..." but then I thought, *Why in the world is his friend not telling him he has egg on his forehead. Does he not notice? Is he too enthralled in his paper?* I couldn't get over this. I decided then and there to always tell people when they have something, such as something in their teeth, or toilet paper hanging, anything, because that is what a friend would do. And why would you be shy to tell a stranger that he or she has a little something there? You are never going to see them again, and it's good karma. You would want someone to tell you.

It is funny, though, if someone notices someone else has a little something. He or she usually just tries to avoid it, look away, and pretend not to see it. Is it that uncomfortable to deal with? And if we are the one with something, it's as if we are embarrassed to get it in front of the person who pointed it out. He or she knows it's there, and now we know it's there. We should be happy that it will not be there now that someone has drawn attention to it. I always tell clients if they have something they may not notice. It lets them know I care—that I am looking out for them. Maybe it is a tag that is sticking out from a client's shirt, or his or her shirt is on inside out; maybe the client has a long whisker on his or her chin. Believe me, he or she is happy I pointed it out.

I started off liking pedicures. We would practice on one another, but when it came time to be out on the floor working on clients, my "like" suddenly began with a "dis." You could say I started to dislike them, despise them really. Did I draw the short straw that I was unaware I was drawing? It seemed that way since I would always get the clients with the bad toe fungus. The ones where the instructor would have to come over and tell them they could no longer come into the school for services, but needed to go see an actual podiatrist.

An older couple came in for pedicures together. I got the gentleman. As I looked at his feet for the first time, I noted to myself to let his feet soak longer than normal. It would then allow me time to either fake an illness or make his feet more desirable, less scaly, and softer, perhaps. Time was up, and I was going in. I tried to find the good in all of it. After all, it was a couple's pedicure. It was sweet they wanted to share a special moment. Nothing says bonding like getting your toenails maintained by a young, starving student with a weak stomach. But as he told me to cut his toenails shorter (and mind you, they were the thickest nails I have ever seen in my life. He could probably climb a tree with his bare feet.) I could not get the clipper to open wide enough to get them over the toenail. So I had to resort to using my file, which took the better half of the appointment. Those were my thoughts, and they were helping take my mind off the situation. His toenails were so tough, I could not make a cut, all while he was yelling at me to dig the white stuff out from under his toenails. One girl walked by as I was working, waiting to be rescued, and told me that I had toenails in my hair. They were the toenails from his wife. They were putting up such a resistance, once they were cut, that they had the power to fly freely. I freaked out, but had to keep it together. I didn't want to touch my hair for fear that white stuff would get on me. What was that white stuff anyway? I went in search of answers, but it was not in my textbook. It was then when the instructor finally came over to evaluate and note that the older man needed a foot doctor. Why didn't he evaluate before I started? That way I would not have to partake in such disgusting jobs that made me reevaluate doing nails in the long run. My nail dreams were shattered very quickly after all I endured. Turns out my stomach was too weak for thick nails harboring white stuff, and there was not enough payment in the world to change my mind.

I had another older lady in for a pedicure. She was wearing stockings. I told her she needed to go into the bathroom to re- move them. She asked if I would go in with her to help her out of them. My answer was no. Again an alarm was going off, and I was wondering where we were getting our clientele. I met her in the pedicure area, where I had prepared a foot bath for her. As she soaked, I told her I would return with the implements I needed for the job. Meanwhile, I was in the dispensary, pointing her out to my fellow classmates, wondering why I got another one such as her. I collected myself and returned, ready to get this behind me. As I worked, she pointed out these bunions. I had no clue what a bunion was. I knew it was that knot on her heel that I was going to avoid! The bad part about a pedicure is that the foot is elevated, your head is leaning down, and there is not much of a gap between your face and the foot. You are all up in the person's foot business. I didn't want to look at a foot that closely. Especially when a bunion needed my attention.

I was getting ready for the massage part of the appointment. She seemed to have fallen asleep. I took this as my cue to slip a towel over her foot so I did not have direct contact. To my luck, she did doze off. I waited a few moments and resumed to the end of the service, where I would apply polish. She mentioned she must have fallen asleep since she couldn't recall the massage. I then agreed with her that she was out, and that she received my full service. When the instructor came over to evaluate, I motioned to her bunions, and again, he told her she needed to go see a foot doctor. This was her last pedicure at our learning school. I walked her to a changing room, but did not help her on with her stockings.

After beauty school, I decided never to do nails again. I was never going to touch another foot. I was never going to look at a foot, let it soak, and try to get through cutting a thick nail all while having others toenails dangle from my hair.

Once I graduated, the world was my oyster. I no longer needed an instructor to check my work. After all, it was no longer my work once an instructor got there. Sometimes they would cut just to cut. I would see what they were holding up, and it would be even. If I had a cute guy in my chair, that was the end of me. It didn't look as if I knew what I was doing. The instructor cut more just to spend more time with the hottie. It was always the cute guy. The main instructor was gay, and he was the worst. He would come over and check forever, hoping he caught something he would have to fix to seem as if he was saving the day; the big hero. My fellow students would talk about how he made up "peeks" so he would have something to cut. Peeks didn't belong. When you pull the hair through your fingers, you check for these spots, blend them, and if it's not blended, the hair will not lay right. I was always good at checking for peeks, leaving nothing to fix. I had to learn to hide my eye rolling with all of the mirrors around, and I did it the hard way. My instructor caught me, confessed he spied me in the mirror. I took notes and realized I took more away from beauty school than just cutting and making sure there are no peeks. Also, make sure you don't roll your eyes at the instructor—who is giving you a passing grade, which will lead to your hair license—when there are mirrors all around, leading you into your future of hair and mirrors.

The day of my graduation was a great achievement, yet such a small affair. It was not as if I had this class where we would start and finish together. We didn't all throw our caps up in the air. When you went to beauty school, you had to have 2,300 hours, so the chances of someone else graduating with you on the same day was rare. So it was a one-man party, with family or whoever could take a few minutes out of their day to come celebrate. Every morning, you had to punch in on a clock, and if you were a minute late, they made you make up fifteen minutes, and that could really add up. At night, you punch out at five o'clock sharp. We would all line up, waiting for the clock to strike, me in my Wendy's uniform, still smelling like burgers. In school, we had to wear white smocks. It was so hard to keep clean, and I only had one, so I was constantly washing it. For some reason, I would get mustard on it every day at lunch. The thing that surprised me was how much hair collected in the pockets. I could stuff a large pillow with all of the hair I accumulated in pockets, shoes, and places you would never believe I would find. But that's in another chapter.

EMBARRASSING TIMES
BEHIND THE CHAIR

I have had many embarrassing times behind the chair, but one moment really stands out. I used to have to take my towels and capes home to wash at night. Once, I took my capes home to wash and some of them had Velcro closures on the neckline. I had other laundry going that night as a mom with two kids does. As I went to work the next day, I placed a cape around my male client, not paying attention since the stylist stationed next to me was talking to me, and when I looked at the neckline to close it, I noticed my thong underwear was stuck to the Velcro, resting on my client's shoulder. I was unsure of what to do at this point, so I started to panic and grab the underwear off the cape while it made that Velcro sound. All along, my client was just sitting there, watching in the mirror, not giving away that he saw it. I was holding it in my hands behind his back, not sure where to put them. I didn't have any pockets, and my station was out in the open with other stylists busy with their Saturday clients, so I threw them in my towel bin.

State Board would have loved that, and I was thankful they didn't usually drop in on a weekend.

I continued on for a moment, ready to go shampoo my client, until I finally burst into laughter and said, "Gosh darn it! I was looking for that pair all morning." I was too. I thought the dryer had eaten them along with one of my socks.

I ended up having to excuse myself to leave for a minute—since my face was clearly red—to go to the breakroom to have a good laugh. I knew he had seen them, since he'd asked why I would need another pair of underwear at work. After it was all over, the next hair appointment he came in for, I told him I could not top that last haircut. It was very memorable. He teased me about it for years, up until he passed.

His daughter got married and I had the honor of doing her hair for her wedding. She came in on her big day telling me what a fun rehearsal dinner they had. They told stories and enjoyed the night, and she said that her dad was especially funny. I asked if he told stories of when she was young. Oh no...He told about the time he'd come in to get his haircut and my underwear had been stuck to the nape of the cape. I still have not topped this, and from time to time, he would remind me that he had seen my underwear. I did get rid of all my Velcro capes, buying only the ones with snap closures.

I was folding clothes one night at home and found a strange pair of underwear. It was definitely women's underwear, but they were not mine. It is a strange feeling when there is an unclaimable pair of underwear in your home, and you don't know how they got there. A true mystery. I went up into my son's room and held them in full expansion, as if they had come to life. He said he didn't know anything about it. Come on! I reminded him they were in his clothes. He finally remembered one of his friends had put them in his coat pocket as a joke without his knowledge, and he found them when he got home. I don't know about you, but it would be curtains if my son put a pair of my underwear in one of his friend's pockets as a joke.

The friend's mom is a client of mine, and I recalled my own embarrassing underwear moment to her. I knew she had a great sense of humor, so I decided to have some fun. I tried to reenact the underwear moment. I folded her underwear inside one of my capes and, when I went to put it around her, the underwear fell out and landed on the floor. I let out a gasp and said, "Oh no! Not again!" Then I said, "Wait! Those aren't mine." She said, "Well they're not mine!" Then I told her she'd better look a little closer. When she finally looked at them, she realized they were hers. I asked her why my son had a pair of her underwear. She said, "Oh yeah, me and your son. Right!" When I told her that her son put them in my son's pocket for a joke, she couldn't wait to get home to talk to her son. I made sure when I went home that night to mention to my son that it would be murder if he ever did that to me.

I did come home one night and could tell that my underwear drawer had been invaded. I was pretty tidy with my drawers, and when I opened it, there was something askew. I also noticed that the necklace holder was moved from my wall and had been placed on the floor of my closet. I yelled for my son to come to my room to see what was going on. He always had a bunch of boys over after school. I called them the smelly boys; I would come home and there they would be, with their shirts off; sitting on my furniture. A smell was in the air when they were there. I could tell the ones who ate fast food because they would smell like old hamburgers. When a teenage boy eats a lot of grease, it just comes out of his pores, and a big dose of cologne will never cover it up.

My son admitted that one of his friends was in my room trying on my necklaces. I asked why he let his friend in my room, and he said he followed him in when he was answering the phone. The friend saw my necklaces and started trying them on. This didn't seem normal. I asked what else he tried on. He said, "That was it." The next day, I went to put a bra on and it had been stretched out so much that I knew someone had tried it on. A woman knows her bra setting and when it has been tampered with. As I was looking for a specific bra, which I never found, I realized I had been robbed. Not only did that boy try on two of my bras but he took one. The most expensive one at that. How do you ask for a bra back from a teenage boy, and do you really want it back? I knew he owed me fifty dollars. I told my son to tell his friend that he owed me. It had been a mystery for a year, and every time someone mentioned this boy's name, I made sure to say that he stole my bra and owed me fifty dollars! A couple of years later, I got a call from the thief. School was out for the summer, and he decided to tell me what happened to my bra. He told me that another boy had taken it. The boy who had put his mom's underwear in my son's pocket. I called this boy's house, and his mother answered. I told her I knew who stole my bra. She asked if it was the original boy. I said it was her son. I heard her holler to her son to ask if he had taken my bra. He claimed it was not him, but I told her to tell him he owed me fifty dollars, that I didn't want the bra back. He still pleaded it wasn't him, so the mystery still lives on.

I guess I have to wonder if I am getting a payback for something I did as a child. Is this karma coming my way? When I was younger, my brother and sister talked me into going into my mom's room to get a bra and a pair of her underwear. We would then dress our dog with these items, filling out the bra cups with her socks and letting him run around our familiar town. Since we lived in a small town, the dogs could run free. There was no dog catcher to worry about, and what if there was? Could you imagine the dog in the back of the patty wagon wearing a woman's bra and underwear? That would be one for the records. I imagined the driver saying to his partner, "Get a load of this," while motioning with his thumb over his shoulder and pointing to the burlesque canine. As it was, everyone knew our dog, so I am sure they drew the conclusion that our dog was wearing my mom's undergarments. Who else could they belong to? The worst part was, when our dog would come home, we would take the items, fold them, and put them back into her drawer. If we put them in the hamper, she would know some-one had taken them. It never occurred to us that the dog lifted his leg a few times and the underwear had to show evidence of his outing.

SIT UP AND UNCROSS

When getting your haircut, if you want it to be even, you need to sit up and uncross your legs. Some clients don't know that by crossing their legs, it throws the balance of their shoulders off and makes the haircut uneven. I am a perfectionist, and I cannot stand an uneven haircut. I guess it is better to have your stylist be type A when getting your haircut. Otherwise, the stylist just might be thinking, *Well, that's good enough. They will never know there's a long spot on the back-left side.* I hunt for that long spot and make it right. Sometimes, the client is ready to be done, but he or she is held captive until I think it's perfect. I had a client in for the first time, and toward the end of the appointment, he mentioned it looked as though it was coming to an end. I said I was almost done and jokingly wondered if he was in a hurry. He then said, "I have things to do. I don't have all day," as he looked at his watch. I let him know I wanted it to be perfect, especially since it was his first time in. I wanted to take my time and really know his hair. It's always best to dry the hair and then detail the cut because sometimes, you do not notice that long spot until you are in the throes of styling.

When I first started out, I worked in a place that charged *à la carte*. The cut was one price, and it was extra if you had anything else besides the haircut. The shampoo was included, but there was a charge of two dollars if you wanted conditioner. It was not ideal if the client didn't want to pay the extra two dollars, if he or she had hair like a scarecrow. It made it hard on the stylist since the conditioner helped close the cuticle down, making it smoother with less tangles. It was hard getting your comb through someone who had long, curly hair, making you feel as if you were wrestling gators. The blow-dry was an extra fee as well. The cheap clients would leave with wet hair, but little did they know, after drying and styling the hair was when I could really put my name on the cut. I could texture it and make sure it was the right length. I would not cut bangs wet since they had a shrinkage problem, so I would dry them first, with no charge.

I have most of my clients trained to uncross when it's time to cut. Sometimes, though, they will start talking and automatically cross, so I then stop cutting and tap their legs. If they don't get what I am trying to get them to do, I give them the look and glance at their crossed legs and then they get it. Other times, I will see them cross, and I will just stop cutting, and the pause will remind them that they have crossed. It is just a natural response for most people to cross.

There are several types of clients who do not sit still. There are the rubber necked ones. You comb through their hair, they relax their neck, and their head follows you and the comb. You then have to hold their head in place with your wrist and lean into them as you comb and cut.

I call the ones who want to look in the mirror to watch what you are doing, the head turners. Reasonable, until I cannot reach them. I turn the chair so my blow-dryer cord will reach them, but they still spot the mirror as if they are dancing, doing a ballet turn. How can a neck turn around so far? The body is facing one wall and the face is still facing the mirror.

You have the leaner. The leaner will be reading a magazine, and his or her head will be lodged forward. If you are standing behind the leaner, you have to have very long arms to be able to reach the top of his or her head. You move the person back to the upright position, but he or she slowly starts to lean again. I think that maybe the leaner doesn't want to look in the mirror; he or she is the opposite of the head turner. Some lean to the left; some lean to the right—so you cannot check for an even haircut. One of my clients knows he is a leaner. He catches himself and comments that he is trying. Another client leans slowly. One minute he's upright, then he gradually is in the leaning position.

I called him a leaner one time, and he replied, "I'm a wiener?" As if I would call anyone a wiener! He was just being funny. He knew what I said and caught himself leaning and straightened up again for a few minutes.

You also have the clients who like to look at you when they are talking to you, so they are a combination of head turners and leaners. They must have eye contact, so they turn to look at me, but I cannot do my job when they are not looking where I put their head. It is best for them to look at me in the mirror while we are talking. Believe me, just because we don't have direct eye contact doesn't mean I'm not listening.

Some clients are just fidgety. Maybe they have had too much coffee and they just cannot seem to sit still. They rock their feet up and down or hit the cape from the inside to knock all of the cut hair off the outside of the cape. Guess where it goes? All over me! If I notice they cannot sit still, I will take extra care to dust them off and blow the hair off from the cape before they go on a hair flying frenzy.

Clients like to read magazines while getting their hair done. I am fine with that. Just as long as they keep their head where I place it and read with their eyes. Some people like to turn their head with each page, as if they are sitting at a tennis match, trying to keep their eye on the ball.

There are the white knucklers. This type of client holds on tight to the arms of the chair as if they were at the dentist. They are afraid of you when you have the shears in your hand. They must think that you are going to just do whatever you want to their hair. This is when I tell them I put the shears in the drawer and am stepping away so we can talk again about what I am going to do. It usually calms their nerves. Usually the white knucklers have long hair down their backs, and their body language is defensive.

They blurt things out, such as, "I'm growing my hair out."

I want to say in return, "Oh, it's out." I mean, how much longer can you have it? It will have to have its own pillow at night, or it could choke you in your sleep. Now there are health hazards we should get into, but they don't want to hear it. I had a client who had colored her own hair, turning it orange. She was in my chair, stressed out and worried about how it was going to turn out after I colored it. I told her she should have been worried when she'd colored it, not when I was going to color it. I always take a moment to reassure them I am well trained.

Some clients try to color their own hair to save money, and then they need to come in to have it fixed, so it ends up costing them more, and then their hair is usually unhealthy from over processing with nonprofessional products. I tell them to, for the next few days, dry-clean only, joking about it to lighten the mood of the frazzled hair, but it is good to give it a rest after all of the recoloring.

I have been to the grocery store, looked down the aisle where the hair color was shelved, and have said to the ladies who were considering a shade, "Don't do it." But they would, anyway, because it said right there on the box what color it would be. Nine times out of ten, it will not look like the lady on the box.

Another one is the Sun-In victims. They usually book their appointments in August when they are getting ready to go back to school. They have orange hair and have clearly spent the summer spraying it in their hair, thinking they will get blonde hair like it shows on the bottle.

The ladies on the bottle, who I doubt use the product, look so happy and inviting. If you have darker hair, let me tell you, it will not deliver. The volume of peroxide is not high enough to lift your hair into a Suzanne Summers. I saw it at the grocery store on the conveyor belt in front of me, next to the purchase separator. I couldn't help myself and asked the lady who the Sun-In was for. She told me it was for her daughter, and I asked what her natural color was. At this point, she was looking at me as if she wanted to tell me to mind my own business, but I felt I had taken an oath with my profession, and I owed it to people like her to tell her the truth. I may squash a few blonde dreams in the summer. She still bought the product, and I wonder to this day how it all turned out and if she covertly wished she would have asked me for my business card.

Let's talk about the ones who cannot keep their hands out of their hair. You are trying to cut, but they have to touch. You put the hair back where you need it, but they move it again and pucker their lips in the mirror as if to see what their hair will look like when it is done. Who actually walks around with puckered lips? I want to know why this is necessary in life. Why don't they see what it looks like when it is done? Sometimes you are drying the hair around the face, and they quickly tuck it behind their ear. You pull it back out to dry it, and they tuck it once again. I wish they made a chair that held clients' arms down to make them sit up the right way, sort of like a straitjacket chair, but then I would not have anything to write about.

I have a client whom I call a bobblehead. He gets to talking and starts bobbing all around. I have to place my hand on top of his head to get him to stop bobbing. By doing this, I am hoping he will get the hint that I am trying to get him to stop, but he doesn't pick up on it. I have had to stop a few times and tell him he is being a bobblehead, and then I mimic his gestures. We both have a laugh, and I think he will stop, but he forgets about it, and bobs some more.

One of my lady clients knits while I do her hair. She has a ton of hair. I cut and weave her color, and it takes longer than the average client. We are spending the better part of the morning together, so she might as well make a hat. Once, she was leaning over, winding up the yarn, and I was chasing her head around. I didn't say anything, but later, as I was drying her hair, she moved suddenly, and I poked her in the eye, knocking her contact out. It was the second time it happened. We did find the contact. It had landed on her cheek. I then teased her about all of the yarn wrapping and pretended to do what she was doing, while leaning forward and off to the side, busy with imaginary yarn. As we both laughed, she said she was going to wear protective eye goggles the next time she comes in.

NO HAIRCUT FOR YOU...
YOU'RE FIRED!

I have the right to fire clients. If I am not respected as a stylist, they are out of here! There are the no show clients who pull the missed appointments; not a favorite of mine or any other stylists. Well occasionally it's OK if it's the last client of the day on a Saturday. Otherwise, I need to charge them. They usually really need in as soon as you can get them in, but I don't feel the urgency, since they so casually blew me off. If they are the habitual ones, and have never compensated me for the time—the time I cannot make up—they are getting the call and are getting fired. Who wants to extend a service to someone who doesn't respect you?

Once I got a taste for this firing, it felt so good to stand up for myself. After firing one client who stood me up all the time, costing me more money than I made when he actually did show, he called me two weeks later and told me he was sorry and that he would pay me for the missed appointment. This was when I realized that just maybe I could train them to behave. He was good for a while, and then one day he called an hour before his allotted time saying it was Tax Day, and he wasn't sure he what he should do; he didn't have time to come get a haircut. I remembered pointing out that it would be Tax Day when I booked his appointment. I asked if he would rather have another day, but he was fine with it. I told him that the choice was his. He could make it to his appointment with me, or just put a check in the mail with the amount of the appointment. He decided he did have time that day to get his haircut after all.

I became the hair Nazi. I started weeding out the ones who did not show. I actually put a mark on their cards displaying that they did not show (N/S!!). These marks go in my client card vault. I have a vault in my mind as well, but if I need proof later down the line, I can pull out their cards and reveal their flakiness. Their cards are for my eyes only, but on occasion I have had to point to that missed date so they know it was documented and I was on to them.

Once this happens—the mark on the card—I know they are flaky, and maybe one day they will want in at the last minute, during a busy holiday when I am already overworked. I may have a list of clients who need in. I will go down the list and put the good client who has never stood me up to the front of the line. I have had a client pay me for his missed appointment and insist I erase the mark on his card so he could have a clean slate. I knew he respected me.

I am famous for saying, "No haircut for you! You're fired. Step aside!" Like the soup Nazi on *Seinfeld*. I tell this to my clients and they laugh, until they miss an appointment.

The number one reason clients use for missing their appointments is that it was on another day, or another time slot. This is an old excuse. Don't use it. It is not true. Another one is that it wasn't in their phone calendar, even though I saw them standing there putting it in. If your phone is acting up that much, then you need a new system! We have a fabulous receptionist who confirms appointments the day before, or sends out a text reminder, so it couldn't possibly be her fault. Also, at the time the appointment is scheduled, she would repeat back the day, date, time, and service. So there is a tip for those who use that excuse. No one is buying it.

Now I work in a salon where I make my own appointments. Clients who don't schedule their next advance times after an appointment text me or call. Every once in a while, there will be a mistype, but I run a pretty tight ship, and I also remind clients the day before. I do hand out business cards with their next appointment as well. Do I really need to pin it to their shirt so they can take it home to their mothers? It can be frustrating since no shows happen in threes. And when I remind the day before, it is just that. It's not a yes or no question: "Can you make it?" It's a confirmation. You have been holding that spot for weeks, and most of the time, I cannot fill it with that short of notice, since my clients are trained to book in advanced since I am usually booked.

I actually have a twenty-four-hour cancellation sign on my mirror, and I joke about writing clients' names under it who have missed appointments with me. I tell them they are the reason for the sign. I have found that if you lose a client, a door opens, and another one comes in. You close a door on a bad client, one who doesn't respect your time, and then there is room for the good client to come through the open door, and this starts a new beginning, making you forget you even have that twenty-four hour cancellation sign on your mirror. I do have mostly nice clients. I have known many of them for so long. I feel like part of their families. I joke with a lady who is somewhat of a saint, and tell her I cannot cut her hair. She asks, "Why?' I then say, "Your halo is in the way."

I fired a client, and a few years later he was back on my schedule. I didn't know how this happened. I asked the receptionist how he had gotten an appointment with me.

She said, "He just called and asked for you, so I put him on your books." Apparently, he had forgotten he'd been blackballed. It is really up to me though, not the receptionist, to tell them they are fired. We really don't have a blacklist by the phone with the names of clients not to book. The only reason this would not work is because when most clients call to make an appointment, they first get the time they want and then say their name.

It would not be good for the receptionist to tell them to hang on, check the list, and say, "There was a mistake. That stylist is booked up for the rest of their cutting days."

I thought I would just leave if he was late, but he showed up early, blocking my only escape route. Sure, the one time I don't want him to show, he does. I made a comment that I was surprised to see him. He told me that the last time he talked to me, I told him he was fired and could never come in again. He seemed to think this was funny. I, however, did not. I have always hated confrontation but have learned over the years to stand up for myself. After all, there he was, in my chair, receiving my services. When we were all finished with the haircut, and he was paying me, he asked if he behaves, if he could come back in. I replayed all of his past appointments. When he would make it, he would say cheesy things to me. One time, while shampooing, he asked me when I was going to let him take me out. Over the conditioner, I said, "My heart is just not in it." He still tried every time to ask me out and just didn't take the hint or listen to my answer. When I fired him, I thought he would get it—that it was never going to happen. I don't know how you could turn it around and think you have a chance of going out with someone after he or she fired you. That is the last statement you say to someone before you think you will never see that person again. If there was a switch to hit, a lever to pull, perhaps, that led to a trap door that sent the person on his or her way, would it then dawn on the person that he or she was not wanted? So *no!* The answer was no; he couldn't come back in. I just squished my nose up as if I was smelling something rotten and told him I didn't think it would be a good idea.

This trap door idea was something to think about. You could have the clients pay up front, ask them where they parked, and when they were bothering you or would not leave, you could hit the correct button to open the trap door and drop them through a tunnel to the south side of the building, where their cars were parked, so you could feel a little accommodating that you didn't make them wander around the lot looking for their cars.

PITA

It's a tax. A tax I charge for the ones who are a pain. You know the ones. They are the ones you see driving or at the supermarket. They have maybe even been through your line. You try to avoid them, but they always come back. You dread having an encounter with them, already knowing the uncomfortable outcome. You wish you could keep them out of your chair and refuse their service.

The only way to feel good about it is to charge PITA. It is a "Pain in the Ass" tax. You raise your price every time they come in, to compensate their rudeness. You tell yourself that it is OK and that you would just charge them extra. This way, the entire time you are working on them, you are thinking how you have a little something on them. You have all the power, and they don't even know it. It makes you seem happy to see them. But you are not. It's just PITA that's making you smile.

I have this one client who's a bit of a pain. Whenever it's time to pay his bill, I already add gratuity in, like restaurants do when you go to dinner in a big group. He is like dealing with a big group: high maintenance, so I need to be compensated. He knows he is looking at the set price. I know I am getting PITA. I have to get PITA, for putting up with the longest forty-five minutes of my life.

He always had to bargain the price, as if it was negotiable. I would tell him the price, and he would lowball me, as if I would just wear down and give in. The thought crossed my mind to just take it, that way he would go, but the sane part of me decided I needed to be paid for what he put me through every five weeks. I wasn't going to reward bad behavior. When you have to reason with your clients as you would with children, they need to pay more. I am not a babysitter.

I told him the market price of the day had just gone up, just like when you go to a fancy restaurant. You want the catch of the day, and maybe it was listed as market price. You are willing to pay because you know it will be good, and you walk in knowing it is going to cost more than the average meal.

I told him. "If you were going to McDonald's, you would pay McDonald's prices, but when you walk into a nicer restaurant, you expect to pay more. I am a nice restaurant. I am not McDonald's. You get what you pay for; so cough it up!" He would rather pay less for the cut and tip more. If the cut was forty dollars, and he gave me a five-dollar tip, it would be forty-five dollars. He wanted me to make the cut twenty dollars so he would give me a twenty-five-dollar tip, which was the same price. But in his mind, he felt better about giving a larger tip.

I said, "If you feel better about giving me a larger tip, then give me a larger tip. The cut is forty dollars." This is why I charge PITA. It is for the ones who are truly a pain.

I had a client who stood me up. I called to remind him of his appointment the day before and left another message that he was twenty minutes late. I ended up leaving thirty-five minutes past the appointment time and was driving to the grocery store when he called. He first apologized for being late, but I corrected him on how he was no longer late after fifteen minutes but that he was a missed appointment. He said he had a hectic day, needed a haircut, and wondered if he could still come in. I told him I was no longer in the salon, that thirty-five minutes was way more than sufficient time to wait for someone who stands me up. He asked if I would come back to cut his hair. I told him I was no longer in hair-cutting mode; I was in grocery shopping mode now, and I was just mentally going through my shopping list. He said that if I came back to cut his hair, he would pay me double. I told him that if he were to pay me double, it just might make me turn my car around. He asked me if he could pay me sixty dollars.

I told him, "No. You usually pay me forty dollars, so it I would eighty dollars. Yes, eighty dollars would make me turn my car around. You better answer quickly, though, because the next left will take me back to the salon, and the left after that will take me to the parking lot of the grocery store." He agreed to pay eighty dollars, so I said I would go back to cut his hair. I returned to the salon, and as I prepared for his arrival, I took a moment to feel proud, knowing that I was worth it.

When he came back to my station, I said, "Show me the money." He said, "I'm good for it." He was.

Another time, he needed in for a cut, and I had been out of town. As I was driving home from my trip, I got the call that he would like to get in the next day. I told him I was booked. He asked what time I would be in and what time I'd be leaving. I told him I was booked from nine thirty in the morning to seven o'clock in the evening and that there was no way I could physically cut his hair after that grueling of a day. People don't realize how hard it is to stand with their arms raised all day, being on. I would challenge anyone to try it for just two hours. It is not for the feeble; let me tell you. He then said he would pay me one hundred dollars. That made me so mad: the fact that I didn't know he was going to ante. I wasn't sure if I wanted to play yet and hadn't even looked at my cards. I just knew I was upset and tired from driving. I told him I was not happy with him, that I would think about it and call him back later when I got home.

I called a friend, and the first thing she said was that she would cut his hair for one hundred dollars. Fine! I called him back and told him I would come in at nine o'clock in the morning for one hundred dollars and to not be late. I got there in the morning, and he was there five minutes early, waiting for me for a change. He said something about the time.

I said, "Don't start with me. I am not on the clock yet." After the cut, I mentioned how nice it would be if he would leave the Living section of the *Oregonian* for me.

He said, "I just paid you one hundred dollars. You can get your own paper." I then reminded him that with my busy schedule, I would not have time to pick one up. He scooped up his paper and left.

It is amazing to me how many people think being a hair stylist is just a light-hearted job. They like to pick your brain about hair ideas on your off time, and say things such as, "I should have asked you to bring your scissors. You could have cut my hair."

I would like to say, "First of all, they are called shears, and secondly, it is my livelihood. I work in my salon, for which I pay rent. I am a businesswoman, and I would not ask you to work on your days off." Think about it.

You have to play hardball, otherwise, they will not take you seriously. Your time is just as valuable as theirs, and once they feel they can take advantage of you, they will do it over and over again. Then you will be depressed that you just put up with it time and again, and you will go home for the day, feeling defeated, with a little bit of your confidence slowly deflating.

SHE WORKS HARD
FOR THE MONEY

Sometimes I do things I don't want to do or deal with unrealistic clients. If I give in and don't listen to my inner whisper, and just say no, it makes me feel I've sold myself short. I then have to resign to the fact that it is now my fault for giving in, and a little piece of me dies inside—until the good things build me back up again. I have a lot of good things, but that's not as fun to write about. At times, the receptionist is like the gatekeeper. Monitoring appointments, trying to supervise who they are, not that she would have any idea. They must appear normal when they call to book the appointment. Besides, it is not her job to screen the clients. I signed up for it. She usually doesn't know they were bad until I come up to her reception area to let her in on what I have been going through with them at my station.

I had a new client in: a middle-aged man. Everyone circling the reception area picked up on his weirdness, but I didn't have a clue until I introduced myself. Then on the walk down the hall to my station, I felt something was amiss with him. My coworkers were all walking by, getting a good look, which made me feel better. At least I wasn't alone, and they sensed a strange bird sitting in my chair. When you have a weirdo in your chair, it's worse when you try to get the attention of your fellow workers, and they are not picking up on your subtle hints, such as throwing hair clips, faking coughs, et cetera. Then you truly feel alone, which is not a good place to be, as if no one in the world knows you have just fallen into a lion's den but you. You try everything but yell names aloud to get the attention of your closest coworkers. Maybe if I could redirect my blow-drying their way. If I were to make their hair move when they were only standing there, cutting, not using any drying features, they would get that I was in distress. What? Do I need to send **SOS** messages your way for you to look over here? Someone…*help*! When you are in that survival mode, a haircut seems to take so long, and you could swear the hair is growing as fast as you are cutting it.

So here I was in my lonely station by myself with this strange man. I was trying to talk to him, give him my service, do the best haircut I possibly could because I am type A and a people pleaser after all, so it was not in my DNA to give a bad haircut to make sure the person would not come back. Usually, you just keep raising the price and hope the person eventually cannot afford you. Again, I was happy the other gals picked up on my discomfort with this guy in my chair, and I didn't feel the solitude. I asked him when he had his last haircut and, without answering my question, he mentioned he was needing a haircut because he was going on a secret mission. Being the joker I am, I asked if he could divulge a little about the secret mission or was it top secret. He just gave me that look. The one that starts to put a little heat on the back of your neck, making your next few questions seem not as important. The usual questions.

"What is your hair history?" Everyone has hair history, yet, they seem caught off guard by this question. You need to know this information. It's not as though I am cracking some secret code of theirs, such as their pin code or something. It can be a number of things. How often they get their haircut, likes and dislikes, how much time they spend styling. This man looked at me as if I was invading his privacy. I was not interrogating!

After that, I moved on, and brought up a new topic. The new topic was yet another one I should have steered clear from. He mentioned he had a new word for the dictionary. One that he's going to try to enlist upon *Webster's*.

He said, "It is not a he or a she."

I said, "You mean like a questionable gender, like a Pat?" Again, he gave me a strange look as if he was wondering why he was talking to me at all. "Like the skit on *Saturday Night Live*?" I added. The look was back, so I thought to myself that maybe I would just be quiet. I couldn't do that, though—not for long, anyway. I felt as though I ran the show, as if I had to entertain. I was on stage, like a stand-up comic in my station. The silence turned up that heat, and the awkward cloud started settling in. Once the cloud hit my station, I was just ready for the client to go. Appointment over. I don't even bother handing out my business card, hoping the person overlooks the cards as he or she leaves, taking his or her money and waving him or her in the direction of the door.

As I was cutting his hair, I noticed two patches of missing hair in the back of his head above the occipital bone.

I told him, "Whoever cut your hair the last time put some holes back here, and I am having a hard time blending them in." He then told me that he cut the hair himself. He needed some hair samples for his secret mission in case something really happened to him. Well I thought something happened to him. He took my business card, said he would come back, and didn't. It left me wondering if something really happened to him, or was that what people said at the end of a new haircut to the stylist to make them feel good? He told me he had a good idea, and that everyone should grow their hair long as a child's. Then they can cut it for a wig, and if they ever lost their hair to an illness, they would have their own wigs waiting for them. This was exactly what made me sleep soundly at night... knowing that one day, due to an illness—if I needed—my hair would be stored in the basement, waiting for me. It dawned on me that this was one of those moments that made me feel as if I'd sold myself out. I almost pointed out right there, "See, your hair does have history. It was now in the basement awaiting a secret mission," but I thought better of it.

As I finished the cut and removed the cape, he asked me to stand right in front of him so he could see my face. Apparently, he was blind without his glasses. Suddenly, I felt less threatened by him and regretted not making obvious gestures to my fellow coworkers so they would be onto my desperate display of dismay. There were clients you would not want to schedule later in the day if you were by yourself. You have to use caution for the ones who gave you that feeling. The feelings that make you want to shutter and look at yourself in the bathroom mirror before you put your smile on and go out to greet them, and sing, "She works hard for the money..."

I was held hostage in my station one day for three and a half hours. Usually, a cut and color takes two and a half hours. This lady had short hair, and she liked to put her hands all in it and tell you how to cut, even jumped out of the chair to look closer in the mirror, while I was in mid-snip. A big time waster. I tried to walk her through step by step, but after a while, I wanted so badly to point out that she was the one sitting in the chair, and I was the one, standing over her with the shears. When I was finally finished, so I thought, I took the cape off, but she always found something else to cut. She threatened to go home and cut it herself. She had me. I didn't want her to go home and cut anything, so back in the chair she went. I tried not to let my face give me away at how unhappy I was. I thought, *I am like Meryl Streep. I could win an Oscar right now.* She had no clue how upset I really was, because now I was acting, but not to the point where I should have given up my day job.

It is upsetting when they question you so much, yet they keep coming back to you, making you feel like a hair God when they love it. You could do it the same way every time, but to them, it is totally different. The same client even had tears. I was thinking they were unhappy tears, but as it turned out, they were tears of joy. My work moved her. Then why was it that when she came in the next time she had to boss me all over again? I then reminded her how she loved it the last time and how she was moved to tears. A little consultation to start was good, but it didn't need to go on for over fifteen minutes. It is so night and day, the feelings they exhibit. You cannot read them one minute to the next. You don't do that to a chef. He creates a masterpiece for you to enjoy, and for some reason you don't like it, you may send it back or eat at another restaurant. I feel as if I am like fine dining. You can tell me how you like it prepared; we can change it around a bit—sort of special order off the side menu, what have you—but if you don't like my menu or the way I prepare it, it is best to go elsewhere.

This lady told me that every time she got her haircut, the stylists told her she could not come back. Gee! I wondered why. When I was finally done, she went off to the bathroom for the final inspection while I swept and waited. And might I add, while I waited, I contemplated that I should charge PITA next time and make a note on her card. I thought about even adding a smile face. When I add a smile face, it has really gotten to me, and I know that I must comply, which, makes me smile.

By this point, I was so exhausted I wanted to cry. They were partially happy tears since I was finally done.

When she left the salon, I looked to the girls who worked across from me and said, "Didn't anyone notice I was being held hostage for three and a half hours?" It is a sad thing when you are at your station with someone and it is not going well, and you look across and feel that no one knows your pain. It's funny when you don't want your coworkers to hear your conversation, and you whisper with your client. That is when they are interested in what is going on in your station, and you have their full attention.

I had an old friend from out of town. I guessed in his mind he thought it was a fantasy to have me run my fingers through his hair. OK, fine. However, I did not see it this way. I did not go to beauty school to one day have this happen, the fantasy, so I could just run my fingers through guys' hair. It was not a dream, nor would it ever be or become some part of a fantasy that I would act upon. It was my livelihood. If I wanted to run my fingers through guys' hair and think I was being erotic, I would have taken up a different profession. I once dated a man who knew I cut hair for a living when we first met. As time went on and he knew how many guy clients I had, he didn't like it. He would ask me, "How many guys' hair did you run your fingers through today?" I didn't stay with him long after that, since his comment was so disrespectful of my profession. I conduct myself professionally, and I take my career seriously, I'm not just some haircutter, hitting on men.

Being the nice person I was, I took my out-of-town friend to my work, cut his hair, and that was that. There was no mention of payment. It became awkward after we got back into my car, since he should have paid me in my place of business, and then it felt weird. The next time he came to town, he mentioned that he really did not need a cut but would not like to miss out on the opportunity for me to run my fingers through his hair again. How did I take this? I didn't find it as a compliment. Once again, this is how I survive. I went ahead and scheduled him. He came in, I cut his hair, and at the end, he said he would take me to lunch. Now, I wasn't sure how to bring the payment up. I felt bad. I should not have felt bad, because this was my business! Holy crap, it happened again! He took me to lunch, but I couldn't eat forty dollars' worth of lunch at the Thirsty Lion. I would rather have my pay and then buy my own lunch, therefore making it less awkward, seeming less like a date.

I really needed to work on this topic of being taken advantage of and the need to become assertive. If anyone else were to be asked for their services, in the profession they chose, they would expect to be paid in full. I could not figure out why it was so hard for me to do the same. It was always brought up in a lightness of ways. Sort of as if it was fun; doing hair was not a real job. I mean, why wouldn't I want to cut someone's hair on my day off or on vacation, since I had the time? They wondered what the big deal was. You don't travel with your shears?

It is the same as asking a plumber, "Where is your snake? Don't you have it on you at all times? I have a clog." Or an actress, "Do something, act. Just turn it on." It's not like that. We all need a break from what we do for a living, and they make you feel as though you would rather die than cut their hair right then.

I went home to visit my family one time and was asked if I could do a perm. Part of me thought I should be flattered they trusted me enough to ask, except for the fact that I was on vacation and did not travel with my perm rods. What about the perm solution? There weren't any beauty stores in the small-town area. Did they want me to go to the grocery store and get a Lilt? I used to use Lilt back in high school. I even thought it turned out well. It gave firm curls, was a bit smelly, but aren't they all? Once I went to beauty school and learned about the different chemicals, I couldn't go back to Lilt! I guess I am a perm snob, and it wasn't the '80s anymore!

I had a new client who lived out of town and was coming to the big city for the weekend with her husband. She liked my profile from the salon's website and sat in my chair with fried blonde ends and black roots. As I tried to work my magic, I found her rather chatty. I just let her talk. It's hard when you realize you have nothing in common and you are trying to connect. Since her hair was so over processed, I had to stay with her and watch her color. It was almost the longest three hours of my life. She was telling me about her grandma passing.

She said, "My grandma died on the shitter!" I was sure my face held a surprised look on it even though I put on my best poker face. She said it again, maybe since I didn't know what to say; she must have thought I didn't hear her. Well I did, and I was hoping the girl in the next station heard her, but as I looked over to her, there was nothing, and believe me, if she would have heard that, it would have gotten her attention. She then said, "She died on the shitter. She had one of those aneurysms from straining, like Elvis."

I jump in with a, "That must have been awful. I'm sorry," to get her to be quiet. When she finally left, I was exhausted. I asked the other girls if they knew what I had been going through for the last three hours. I then said, "Did you hear what happened to her grandma?" They didn't have a clue. "She died on the shitter," I said.

Sometimes when I am working hard on one client, if he or she is high maintenance or has enough hair for two heads of hair, I stop and put my arms down and tell the person I need a rest, and then I dance around him or her and sing, "She works hard for the money...so you better treat her right."

THE CLIENT CARD BOX

My client card box is my vault. It holds so much history. I write down when the client has been in, every time he or she has been in, so if the client is due, I call him or her and do some recruiting. Sometimes I will look up the clients I am not that excited about coming back, and will celebrate a little if a few months' time has lapsed, knowing they must have had it cut already and were well into a hair affair in some else's chair.

I write color formulas down on the clients' cards and make sure they like what I did. I never just get the card out, knowing they will be in, and mix. Until I see the whites of their eyes, I never mix. That would be the one time they wouldn't show or they would want to change their color formula a little. I occasionally write a note if they have been difficult. Maybe it would be time to start charging them PITA. Maybe I would give them a few strikes first. It would depend on my mood they put me in with their mood. Clients will text me, saying they are on their way, and I will text back, asking if they want the same color, so I can mix the color. Most of the time, they do, so I will then set up and be ready when they walk in, and I see they were late because they stopped at Starbucks.

I worked with a girl who wrote everything about them down on the clients' card. The way they liked their coffee, if they were taking any vacations, their kids' names, and birthdays. I started doing that as well, but then I realized I could remember those things without notations. I know all of my clients' birthdays, their spouses, and some of their kids. I have a memory for dates and have all of my clients' birthdays in my head, and I call to sing to them on their special day, making up corny songs that either rhyme with their names, the dates, or their ages. I know most of them appreciate it, because if I get busy and sing later in the day and they answer, they will wonder what happened to me. If I forget all together—if I get really busy at work—it makes me feel terrible. I have started something and once they are pampered in that way, they look forward to it each year. Sort of like a dessert that comes with the meal: a little bonus.

Once in a while, a client will ask to see his or her card. Never let them see the card! It is for your viewing only, like at the doctor's office. Do you ever get to see your chart? No! So I usually study it before they arrive and tuck it out of their reach, and then I am careful to put it back in the drawer so it's not left out for their viewing. You know if they see their card, they will naturally want to look at it. I then hide it under the stack of foils or in a drawer. If you take the time for them to see you putting the card back into the vault, they may ask to see it. I have, on occasion, scanned to see if I wrote any notes about them and flash it to them quickly. Remember, it is your vault and only you have the key.

I have a client who grabbed his card and was reading it while I was washing out a color bowl. I came back and saw him reading his card. He asked me what all of the marks (recut!!) were about. I told him he went through a recut phase for a while and that I would mark it on the card.

"I wanted to make sure I cut it shorter so you would not have to come back again." My real answer was that I was getting ready to charge him for taking up two haircut spots and only paying me for one. Sometimes two weeks would go by, and then he would call and say he needed more off. There's that old joke about how a bad haircut will look good in two weeks, since it has had time to grow. If hair grows a half an inch a month, then that is a fourth inch I'm not getting compensated for, so I'm marking it on his card.

Another mark I put on client cards if they don't show is *N/S!!* I always use two exclamation marks. It is more dramatic that way, and sometimes, when I have to start charging them for their missed appointments, since they are repeat offenders, I will show them their cards and point out the dates they didn't show. They know I have them then.

THE GHOST

You weed through your client cards, notice the clients who have not been in for a while, and you throw their cards away. For some reason, they must feel this, and they call. They are on your schedule, and they want to know the last time they were in. You don't want to tell them you threw their card away, so you pretend to look for it in your file, maybe even claim to see it, and you, purport to peek at the date and quickly put the file away.

I am so lucky. I can usually search my brain and find something there to jog my memory, like the time of the year perhaps, or someone's birthday, and the date will just come to me. I do know this happens, though. If there is a client you want to see, just throw his or her card away. Somehow, he or she will feel it and that client will call. I have held onto the ones I am not that excited about seeing, though...just to make sure.

I saw a client years after he had moved away. I threw his card away, since he had not been in for years and had moved out of state. He asked me when was the last time he was in with me to get a haircut. I told him I didn't know; I threw his card away. He had that puzzled look on his face as if he was appalled that I would do that to his card. He just said, "You threw my card away?" See, he came back, and now he has another card in my file.

I cannot bring myself to throw away the cards of the clients who have passed. I keep them at the back of the alphabet and feel a little melancholy as I am leafing through the cards.

RECRUITING

Sometimes, during the slow season, you may have to call a few clients and recruit them to come in. You try to sound all official, and they may think the dentist office is calling. You lower your voice and say, "My records indicate that it is time for your next visit. Report to me ASAP."

You just know they are going to call the following week when you are booked solid, and want in, so you will beat them to it. We all know that when you think of a client, within the day or two, he or she will call and be on your schedule. Why not use that ESP and get them in?

I had the dreaded two-and-a-half-hour cancellation in the middle of the day and wanted to fill that gap, so I recruited. Clients tell me to call them when I have no shows and gaps in my schedule, but when there is a no show, I usually wait for fifteen minutes, call them, and then find out I had time, but not always enough time to recruit. Most clients love when I call them to get them in. They know I am thinking of them, and it makes them feel special.

Everyone should know by now that I will only recruit the good clients, the ones who respect my time.

I have one client whom I call every month to recruit. I just know he will want me to stay late another night, and this way, I can offer a few time slots, or put him within my scheduled working hours. One day, I called and told him I would be out of town the following week and knew he would be due for a cut. I told him he could come in the next couple of nights.

He said, "What about tonight? What time are you done?" I told him I didn't have any openings tonight, and I didn't offer any; I was working until 6:45 p.m.

He said, "Well, it would work best to come in at 6:45 p.m."

Again, I said, "I'm not offering tonight. I have tomorrow or the next day open." He mentioned again how it would be best to come in tonight. I then told him that I had seven haircuts scheduled in a row, and that he would not want to be the eighth! We finally scheduled for the following day after what felt like a Laurel and Hardy shtick. Then at 6:40 p.m., the receptionist came to my station to tell me he was in the lobby, and he wanted to buy some mousse. I could see right through this one. I was not falling for it. I had cut his hair for several years now, and he had never purchased hair products from me before. He wanted me to come to the reception area so he could ask me again about staying late to cut his hair, never minding the fact that I would be so hungry that I would have passed out. I thought that if my stylist was hungry or tired, I wouldn't want her to operate her shears around my head.

I told the receptionist to tell him that I would love to help him pick out a mousse tomorrow night at his scheduled time. The next night, when he came in, I mentioned that I knew what he was up to.

He then said, "I needed some mousse." The man did not need mousse! He didn't have that much hair. I ended up showing him a nice product that would keep his flyaway hairs at bay, and he bought it that night; I thought he did it to show he was sincere in his product needs the previous night. Give an inch, I tell you, and they will take a mile.

A couple of years later, I moved to Sola Salon Studios, and I had my own retail displayed for clients to purchase. I mentioned to him that I had a few different product lines, and if he wanted, I could pick out a few products that would work for his hair.

He then said, "I don't need no stinking mousse!" That brat.

I truly enjoy the fun banter I have with my bratty clients. It keeps me on my toes, and entertains them.

Actually, to clear things up, I have way more good clients than bad. The bad ones just stick our more, like a thorn in your foot. You are standing there, trying to cut their hair, but there is that thorn. The more you do their hair, the more the thorn gets embedded into your sole. Soon it is a part of your foot, like the clients' cards is part of your file...and there, it remains.

THE HAIR AFFAIR

I t happens, the hair affair. I have been the one the client is having the affair with and I have been the one my client has the affair on. Either way, it is awkward.

I once had a client who was going to have an affair with me. She called to ask me if I was good. Good enough to leave her current stylist for. She didn't want to have the affair and regret it as well, if I wasn't worthy. Besides, what was I supposed to say? "I'm terrible. I really don't know what I am doing, and I really don't want to be the 'other' stylist." I knew I was going to have to work at winning her over, since she was questioning me over her current stylist—whom she was not happy with—or she would not be calling me. She ended up being very happy with my work and left the former stylist for me. I did her hair for years, until one day she came in to tell me that she was going to go to beauty school. I told her that she was my client and couldn't do that. She couldn't leave me for all that experimental learning in the school of beauty.

Well she did, and one day, she accompanied me to a hair show. I couldn't believe I was sitting there in the class with her. It was as if you decided to become a doctor, and then you were sitting there with your doctor, learning new techniques, after he or she had seen you naked. It was a feeling that she shouldn't be behind the scenes. I kept forgetting that she was now, just like me, working in the hair professional field. She was very happy and successful, and it was gratifying to know that I influenced her in a way that made her want to do what I was doing. It was hard to let her go, though. I held onto her client card for a long time, with all of her color formulas and the dates she had come in for services, even though I should have thrown it away, in hopes that she would return to my chair.

She used to come in and bring little film canisters with her, so she could take some color home with her to dye her "lower re-gions," since this was not one of my menu options. There was no guessing that she wanted to be anatomically correct. The first time she did her own coloring and showed her husband, he said, "Did Debbie do that?" Right! Like I was going to partake in something so personal, so far off course where I would have had to leave my station and find a private space to accommodate such a service. Besides, I waited until pajama/tickle parties for the hair coloring fun to begin. Just one of many things women do at these parties that men fantasize about. I offer services that I can do openly at my station with coworkers and clients walking by. One day, I saw the husband and mentioned that his wife had been in to see me. He asked if she got some color. What could I say to that? I was starting to turn red at the idea that I was the one matching the curtains to the drapes. I just nodded and left it at that.

I think it is politically ethical to only work on parts that are exposed above the cape. The neck is included, but could become questionable the hairier the guy. Sometimes, the guy is so hairy you wonder, Where do I draw the line? If the hair is well below the neck of the cape, I put a towel down in the neck of the shirt as far as I can, and I use the clippers to clean the neckline. It is just that though, a neckline…not an upper back line. There is no need for anyone to remove his shirt. Back in the day, when I was starting out and would do a few kitchen cuts, I had a guy who would come to me, and he would always take his shirt off. I wasn't sure if he was thinking he didn't want cut hairs on his shirt, or if he was trying to show off his physique to me. It was awkward when he walked into the bathroom to check out his cut, and he had me take off the cape, and leave the room half-naked.

I try not to cut the neck hair in a straight line, but rather sculpt it in a scoop, upside-down moon sort of thing, following the line of the collar. Once, I had a man so hairy, I did just that, but as I cut, the other hairs under the cut-off line were like wild vines, stretching toward the sun and escaping under the collar of the shirt. I sort of just brushed them down and pulled the shirt up over them. This is where a blow-dryer can come in handy. You can use the force of the air to blow the back hair back down where it belongs. If you are brave enough, you can give the client a referral to the lady who waxes. It did strike me a bit odd as I saw the shirt protruding, not even resting on the guy's skin on account of the padding of the hair supply.

It is hard to see your client sit in another chair. Really, we are happy to see you. We are happy you stayed in the salon, and we do get over it, but it may take some time. It is not the other stylist's fault. Sometimes, the client just needs a change or clicks better with another stylist. It is hard not to take it personally.

I had a client come in who was going to another stylist in the salon where I worked. He worked two stations over, so we were not hard to miss. She would sneak in to get her bangs trimmed with me on his day off. One thing led to another, and she decided to take it to the next level of cutting and coloring, having a full hair affair. We had made an appointment for her to come in on the other stylist's day off. We thought we were being sneaky, but the other stylist came in to get something, and there we were, my hands in her hair. We were caught! We felt bad, but it was sort of a relief that we were out in the open. No more sneaking around for our afternoon hair rendezvous; we could just be in it now, without all of the guilt. Well, I had some guilt, because I had to talk about it with the other stylist so we could move on. We are still together, nineteen years and growing strong.

It was harder to get her husband to join me, though. Every time we made an appointment for him, the other stylist would see him on my schedule, call him, and move him back to his books. The client felt bad, so he would just stay. Then the day came. I knew he was coming in under a fake name. I was stressed out about being caught and didn't want the other stylist to be mad at me. It was scheduled on the other stylist's day to work as well, so we were being brave. The stylist saw him in my chair and chose to ignore him. I guess what I am getting at is that we do not own our clients. They have the right to come in to see who they want, guilt free.

I have to admit that I secretly think clients must have passed away when I have not seen them in a while. Death would be the only reason they were not back in my chair. Otherwise, they would be here, having me do their hair. I check the obituaries to see. I am glad I do not see them there but cannot for the life of me figure out why they left me.

This is the biggest mystery one will never solve. It can be years into this cutting relationship, and then one day the client drops off the face of the earth. You are left to recap the events from the last time he or she was in your chair, looking for clues of his or her unhappiness. Was it something I said, or did? Maybe something I didn't do? It must have been my fault, or else they would have been back. You spend some time beating yourself up over it. I guess hair stylists are insecure. We take things personal, like an artist who has unsold art. It is just business, yet somewhat personal since we spend so much time getting to know our clients.

It would be nice to at least get a note explaining why clients decided to leave. That way, your self-esteem does not have to suffer. Sometimes I dream and pretend to win the lottery. I ask myself if I would keep my day job. The answer is always the same. I would keep the clients I enjoy. The ones who I think rely on me and cannot live without me. I cannot imagine not seeing so-and-so. Then one day, so-and-so is gone, and you didn't win the lottery and are left to ponder and search the obits once again.

I have a client who only has me highlight her hair. She goes to another stylist, in another salon across town, for her haircuts. She was telling me about how hard it was to go to two different salons, and that the other stylist always cuts her bangs too short. I told her that I cut hair as well as doing the color, and I have a strict policy never to cut the bangs too short. Originally when she came to me, the stylist who did her color had a stroke, and she went to another stylist for her haircut. When the other stylist who cut her hair retired, she never asked who was going to cut her hair, she just went out and found another stylist to cut it and still came to me for the color. She said it never occurred to her to just come to me for the whole appointment. So for her next appointment, we booked a haircut and weave, but I did give her an assignment. I told her she had to send her other stylist a note explaining why she was not going to see her anymore for her services. That way, the other stylist could save herself the whole thought process while keeping her ego intact, instead of having to search the obituaries.

She did tell me one day that she ran into her former stylist who cut her hair, and all she could say to herself was, "Thank you, Debbie, for making me write to this lady." She said it made it less awkward since she had been so kind in her note.

If one of my clients had to have a hair affair on me, I'd usually ask them a series of questions:

1) Who was he/she?
2) How did you meet him/her?
3) Did it mean anything?
4) I'm sure you were thinking of me the whole time, right?

Well, my questions are usually answered because they are back in my chair. I usually know right away if they have had an affair since I know how long they go between cuts, and I can tell my own work. They are not fooling anyone, and when I say anyone, I mean me.

THE BLAME

I have several clients I have had for years. They started coming to me when I was just starting out. They were young, I was young. Now, they are getting older, as we all are, and they may have some gray hair. They like to blame me, since it has changed over the years while in my chair. They tell me they didn't have any gray hair until I started cutting their hair. I think this is funny. It's not my fault, and if I really had this power, do you think I would be cutting hair? Do they really believe this? I guess they would rather blame me than face the fact that nature is taking its course, taking it as a cue to explain the hair coloring options I have to offer them.

I told one guy, after listening to him blame me for his gray, that when he started coming to me, he was young. Now he was a grandpa, and that was why his hair was gray. It was really not my fault, but he loved to argue with me about it. He knew I would not take the blame. Thinning hair clients are the same. It is hard when they ask you if their hair is getting thinner. What do you say without making them feel bad?

"No. I will always have a job cutting your hair." Sometimes, when you realize they do have a lot less hair than they used to, you feel badly about charging them full price. Would it make them feel worse if you told them they were getting a discount because they didn't have the head of hair they used to have? If they were looking for a bargain, I guess they would go to the barber shop down the street called the Donut Cut. It actually says on the sign BALDER IS CHEAPER. See, even balding people love pampering.

I had a client come in who had a stray hair in the middle of his forehead. I pointed this out to him since he was sort of a brat, and I felt the need for him to notice it. He asked me why there would be a hair in the middle of his forehead.

I told him, "That is where your hairline used to be. Now, it is receding, and that is the last hair that is left from your original hairline." I had to keep a straight face with my line delivery, suppressing my laugh, but the look on his face made it hard. He asked me to tweeze it. I told him there would be a tweezing fee. I got out some tweezers and pulled it out. He did lay an extra ten dollars down after the haircut, but I thought it was for missing an appointment a few days ago, and he actually owed me more for standing me up. The next time he came in, he told me he had overpaid me ten dollars.

I told him, "That was for the tweezing fee." Now, when he comes in, he asks me if that hair is back and makes some comment on how it's ten bucks a pluck!

The same guy with the receding hairline and the one stray hair I most often leave—on account of his pocketbook—wanted to know if his hairline was getting worse. I decided to get my tape measure out to see. I measured it and took note of it on his client card that was in the vault. A couple of years later, he asked me if his hairline was getting further back. I got out the tape measure again to see, and checked the notes on his card from the first measure. It had receded slightly. Now, every new year, he has me measure and record it on his client card. I told him he would have to start growing his eyebrows longer and comb them back since his hairline was going that way as well, that it would soften his forehead.

Another client I've seen for haircuts for over twenty-six years mentioned his receding hairline. He said it used to not be so bad. I waited for him to blame me, but he didn't. It had receded on both sides in the front. He said it was like a double car garage, and you could park two cars in there. One day, I found a stray hair in the bare zone and pointed it out to him, as I feel it were my duty, so when I cut it off, he would not be left in the dark. He asked what that hair was and why it was there. I told him it was the parking attendant. We both laughed, because he was the one who mentioned his double car garage. As time went by, and it receded further back, he said his double car garage was leading to the big parking lot, since his hair was thinning on top.

Clients also like to blame you when their grey hair starts showing through the hair color. Hair does grow! It is a scientific fact, and it is a good sign you are healthy. We cannot prohibit the rate of hair growth, just as we cannot make it grow. Hair grows about a half an inch a month. In two weeks, you will start to see some grow out. This is not a news flash. It's just like kids who like to put the blame onto others.

Instead of just owning up to it, they are fast to say, "It wasn't me." I had a lot of this going on at my house when my kids were young, and never wanted to take the blame. One night, I found a pork chop behind the bookcase in the dining room.

When I asked my kids whose it was, they both said, "It wasn't me." Well, I knew for a fact it wasn't me, so it had to be one of them. I found another one in a vase, stationed on the table, wrapped in a paper napkin, under the artificial flowers. Wasn't Me was so busy in my house, so as I set the table one night for dinner, I set an extra place setting. As we were all around the table, my kids were both asking who was coming to dinner.

84

I said, "Wasn't Me." They looked at me as if I had a horn growing out of my forehead. I continued, "Wasn't Me has been so busy around the house, I figured he was hungry. He threw the pork chops behind the bookcase and in the vase; he wrote on the bed spread..." And I named a few more things to make the point of why Wasn't Me must have been starving. They did not find the clever humor in it, and after that, Wasn't Me moved on.

I have a balder gentleman who comes in. One time, he went for over two months without a haircut. He had a few stray hairs on the top of his head that I clipped off. Otherwise, it would look as if he were trying to get a TV signal. You wouldn't want ten lone hairs on the top of your head to grow out. You wouldn't be able to easily get them to lay down. They would want to stand straight up. If there are fewer than twenty hairs up there, or only one hair, per square inch, it is best to just get rid of them. That is not enough for any coverage and only draws more attention to the fact that there are only ten hairs on top, so it is my duty to make sure my clients are walking around looking groomed. Again, I took an oath. Besides, a groomed head looks better than one trying to keep the last bits just because it can. I told him it had been at least two months since he had been in. He thought it had only been one month. I held my comb up to a single erect hair on his head, using the ruler on my comb to read the diagnosis.

I said, "It is an inch, so it had been two months. That's a half an inch a month." There was nothing more he could say. He's a very smart man. He gets it. I love that I can tease with my clients, and I hope no one takes it the wrong way.

One time, as I was walking a man to the shampoo bowl who didn't have much hair, I heard a little boy say to his father, "Look, Daddy. That man is running out of hair." I quickly started a conversation as to distract from the situation.

Most clients have a normal size forehead, which is, in truth, a four-head. This type of forehead looks good with or without bangs, depending on the shape of the face. Some, who are receding or have a bigger space there, I call a five-head. It is taller than a four. This type of forehead looks better with bangs or a soft fringe to not appear so bare, sort of like a big picture window. When you add a curtain or some blinds, it takes away from the nakedness. Then you have the three-head. It is best to not have bangs. Bangs on a three-head would be like trying to fit furniture from a two-bedroom apartment into a studio. It shortens the face, and then it looks as if your hair is wearing you, instead of the other way around.

I was blamed for an entirely different reason one afternoon, other than causing gray hair or baldness among my longtime clients. It was Easter time, so I had my candy bowl out, filled with chocolate foil-wrapped eggs. I told a guy who came in to wait for me at my station. As I got to him, I noticed he had a chocolate egg he was starting to unwrap. I put the cape on him, figuring he could unwrap it after the cape was on, then I proceeded to cut his hair. After the cut, I took him to the shampoo bowl; the chocolate egg was not on my mind. When I was all finished with him, I dusted him off and removed the cape. At that moment, I saw he had chocolate melted all over his shorts and partly on his shirt. I asked him what happened to his clothes. He looked down and then said he didn't know; it wasn't there until I put the cape on him. Another reason they should keep their hands above the cape, where I can see them. As if I have chocolate on my capes, and it was my goal to spread it on my clients. I told him I only used one cape per client, and I washed them after each use, so there was no way the cape had chocolate on it. I then saw the half-melted chocolate on the floor, under the chair, and pointed it out to him. I remembered he had one with the green foil wrapper, and that was what was on the floor. He had no idea how good of a detective I was and that I paid attention to the small details. I asked if he ate the chocolate he had in his hand, that he was unwrapping when he first got to my station. Then, thinking about it, I didn't recall him ever eating it. So he must have just held onto it while it started to melt, so he dropped in on the floor, but for some reason, he was blaming me. I watched as he left and got into his girlfriend's car. They were having a long conversation. I wondered if she was asking what happened to his clothes. I pictured him telling her how I had chocolate on my cape, and that it got all over his clothes. It was the strangest thing that he didn't own up to his own chocolate disaster. That was the last time I ever saw him. After ten years in my chair, chocolate came between us. Either he was too embarrassed, or he really thought it was my fault. But I would not take the blame.

THE SUPPORT GROUP FOR THE BANG TRIMMERS ANONYMOUS

You have a client in, and you already know she cut her own bangs the moment you greet her. You honestly don't believe the rest of the hair can grow—while the bangs stay the same, not growing at all—or the bangs seem shorter than the last time you saw them. You just know the client will come clean when you get near that part of her hair. Finally, you are in her fringe area, and she blurts her confession out. You tell her you already knew it was she who did the damage, and you point to your hair license on the wall, reminding her of why you have one and she does not. You tell her to hand over the kitchen scissors, or the Swiss Army Knife, and report to the twelve-step Bang Trimmer's Anonymous. The class for self-cutters, bang trim abusers.

In the class, there is a circle of short fringed ladies, and they are talking about their haircutting mishaps. The self-inflicting ones. It goes something like this:

"Hi. I'm Martha."

"Hi, Martha."

"I have been a bang trimmer for about two years now, and I cannot help myself. I am an embarrassment to my family and my hair stylist, but I just cannot stop," says Martha.

The bang trim abusers inadvertently look around the circle as they plead their stories and notice a lady who really went to town and wonder what her story was. Everyone excitedly hopes she shares. Members divulge their weakest moments, maybe because of a bad night's sleep and then waking up in the morning, hoping for second-day hair, and it just wouldn't lay down right. They got the scissors, knowing the outcome, but they were possessed. They must cut, just a little. Enough to get them through the day, but they always take it to that next level. The level of the obvious self-trim. They end up having to walk around with their eyebrows raised just to close that gap between their eyebrows and the bottom of their bangs. People think they look surprised, or perhaps, wonder if they have had too much coffee.

Nothing helps their bangs grow when they are waiting for a miracle, even pulling on them. They just have to wait it out and remember what that feeling was like, to keep themselves from being repeat offenders. They read articles on how to speed hair growth, then wonder how they can just target certain areas. They try their round brushes, but the bangs are too short to fit around the brush, and now they are sticking out, more noticeable and angry. They try pinning their bangs back, but they look so bare, like a peeled onion. They think to themselves, *It will be another bad bang day. I need help!* They Google the bang trimmers support group in their areas.

After they share their stories with the group, they will have to get sponsors and call them when they have cutting urges: "I have the scissors in my hand right now. I am in the bathroom mirror, and I am going to do it." The sponsors will have to talk them out of it and tell them to put the scissors down. They will even meet one another when needed, because they too have been there, but their bangs are now fashionable.

One of the steps in the program should be to actually grow the bangs out, to not have them anymore, or the urges that come with having bangs. Not good if you have a tall forehead. Tall foreheads need a little softening, even a swooping side bang to ease the bareness a big forehead can portray. Bangs are not easy to grow out. It is the one spot that seems to take the longest, like its growth has been stunted there somehow. I tell my clients to make their hair grow faster, they should stand on their head every night for five minutes. They always believe what I say, knowing I have hair knowledge. They want a five-minute miracle to believe in. When their bangs are all grown out, they have done it, and now they can become sponsors.

Then you have the clients who love to cut their own bangs; they prefer it. The haircut is perfect, but then, there are those bangs. They are the first thing you see. It's hair by Debbie, bangs by Martha. I cannot take credit or be responsible for bangs cut too short. I had a client who wanted the really short bangs. I just could not bring myself to do it. I guess it stems from being a child and having my mom cut my bangs. I would always sit so still, and yet they would always end up on a slant. I guess it scarred me. The client went home and cut her own bangs very short, giving herself baby bangs. The kind that curve up in the corners, like they are smiling. The kind that, if they really are necessary, should be on a six-year-old with a jump rope.

There are a few clients who come in, and I don't detect the self-bang trim right away. Later I will notice a hole and think to myself, *I don't drink and cut, so what happened here the last time I cut this hair?* That is not my work. I ask, and they admit that they did it. I have clients who tell me they did it when they were drinking. This is something I just do not get. Were the bangs hanging in your martini or getting caught on the little umbrella? Then why cut them in that circumstance? Why not wait until you have sobered up? People get the strangest ideas when they are drinking. Maybe they are attending the wrong support group.

When I am done cutting their hair, I will have a client ask me to cut the bangs shorter. I will just take a little more off, sort of just go through the motions. They will ask me to take more, and I'll think they will be too short, and I wouldn't want to do that to anyone. I wouldn't want anyone hating me for cutting their bangs too short because I would not be able to sleep at night. It is my number one fear, besides spiders. If they want them any shorter, I will have them sign a waiver claiming they were the ones in control of this big decision. It is my insurance, and I will be making a claim.

It is not as easy as it looks, cutting bangs. Some clients say they have been watching me do it, that it doesn't seem that hard, so they will just barely cut them, but something always goes wrong. Some clients will cut them when they are wet, not allowing for the shrinkage to occur. Others will cut more into the bang area, taking away from the sides. Back in the '80s, this was acceptable. It was a pie-shaped bang, a big triangle in front. A slice of pie, I like to call it. I tell them if they want a slice of pie to go to a cafe. It is best when the bangs blend with the rest of the hair. A slice of pie does not blend. It is hard to grow that out when they do this to themselves. I then tell them to step away from the scissors.

I have a client who always takes chunks out of her hair. I asked her what she used to do this fine job. She told me she used her husband's nose hair scissors. I usually know when she is due for a cut and try to call her and get her in before she does too much damage. The kind you cannot recover from for quite some time, like the early thaw when the groundhog comes up and then runs for cover. One day, she called me and wanted in. I told her I was surprised she was needing in so soon. She told me she and her husband were trying a temporary separation, and he obviously took his nose scissors, so she was in need of my services. I felt bad for her that she was going through a hard time, but happy for her hair for getting a rest from scissors that had recently seen the inside of a man's nose. They are back together now, so it's around-the-clock worry.

I had a male client who was in. As I neared his ear area, I noticed a big chunk of hair missing.

I asked, "What happened here?" He said he thought it was too long and just wanted to take a little off to get by. Now, I could have just let him off the hook without asking more questions, but I needed to get to the bottom of this compulsion that part of my clientele had. I noted that the other side remained intact, from what I had done on the last haircut. I asked, "So what did you think when you saw what you had done?"

He said, "I looked at it and said *oops*." Again, I asked what was going through his mind when he saw the wreckage and the hair that probably lay in the sink. He said he knew then that he shouldn't try cutting the other side and to call to schedule an appointment the proper way. So this support group is now coed.

I had a roommate during beauty school who had the curliest hair. When it was wet, it would just kink up, all the way to her scalp. With some time, she would dry and curl it, leaving me amazed at how far she could make it stretch. She never went to a hairdresser. It really didn't grow much. It would just break off from all of the hot tools. At times, when a strand was not cooperating, she would just cut it off. When in doubt, cut it out was her motto. I would find all of these little dark curly hairballs lying around in the bathroom. The first time I saw one, I didn't know what it was. As I began to scream and it lay motionless, I realized it was either dead or in no way able to harm me. As I poked it, it dawned on me it was a clump of hair. I asked my roommate about this morning ritual she had going. She told me that if she was doing her hair, and there was a piece that was not doing what it should have been doing, then she was cutting it off. Visually, I tried to scan her head, looking for obvious digits, signs of her self-cutting, but she had me. Her curling iron was doing some great cover up work. There was nothing in my textbook about this.

The number one rule for bang trimmers: never cut them when they are wet. They will shrink. Also, don't tape them down, thinking you will cut a straight line at the bottom of the tape. If you have a cowlick, it won't be straight. The number two rule: don't think you are going to take cutting notes from what I am doing and go home and try to replicate it. I am standing above you, a trained professional, and my scissors are shears, and I use them only for cutting hair. The most important rule is: just don't cut them. Hide your scissors from yourself. If you know you are having friends over for a few glasses of wine, or you feel your bangs are at that "in your eyebrow too much zone," just hide them. Maybe use the buddy system. Trust your friend to hide your scissors from you in your weakest moment. If you are in that moment of cutting them, just dial my 911 number, or text me, and I will gladly squeeze you in.

THE CASKET CUT

There's a guy client I have had for twenty-nine years. I was so young when he started going to me for his haircuts. I used to always cut my finger while doing his hair. Maybe since my shears back then where cheap and his hair was too thick to get through. Or, I needed to sharpen the cheap shears once a month, who knows.

"I was still wet behind the ears," he used to say to me. He started going to me after his male hair stylist got sick.

The stylist told him, "Debbie may be new to this, but you are going to love her and be with her forever." I never knew that part, until years later. He was right.

He likes to blame me for the gray hair he has mainly in the front.

He calls it, "His foreign hair, not gray." He said he didn't have any when he started coming to me, that I caused it. I tell him that when he started coming to me, he was young, as I was. Now, he was an old grandpa. This always got him, made him a little snarky. I told him I felt a few gray hairs popping out on my head, due to the stress he caused, and that was why it was best to be a blonde, to easily hide the gray ones.

He told me that when he died, before he was buried, I was going to cut his hair one last time! I always told him there was *no way* I would *ever* do a casket cut! He told me that if it was in his will, then I would have to do it. We usually fought about this for a while each time he came in. Sometimes, I looked at the clock and noted that it only took four minutes for him to bring it up. The subject came up upon every appointment. Other times, I was surprised that we almost made it to the end without its mention.

I weighed my options. He had a lot of hair, so I would be in business with him for some time. He did not stand me up, so he would not be fired. I may very well be put into this position. I forever told him that it would never happen and tried to change the subject. He loved to argue over this, since he knew it freaked me out. I couldn't imagine cutting his hair after he has passed, but he forced me to picture it. I wondered what it would be like. Would there be background music to soften the mood? Would I feel awkward and just start talking, bringing up old times? What if I got creeped out? Would there be someone I could give the shout out to who would come running, to fill my comfort? These were thoughts I started to realize were not normal.

After a few discussions, I told him I might just do it to get the last word in with him. Maybe I would do something funky to his hair before he was laid to rest, such as a Mohawk or the dreaded mullet. I would definitely put some thought into this. After all, I only had to cut the front and sides, since the back would not be seen.

I told him this and he replied with, "Oh no. You will have to cut it the way you always cut it." I told him he would be lying down, so I would not be able to get to the back of his head.

He then told me, "They will have me propped up so you can get the back. I am going home today and will take a picture of how it is now, and the picture will be there, so you will have to cut it like the picture."

OK, who thought like that? And if they did think like that, who said it aloud? Gross. On my station, I had a wooded hand that held my business cards. I told him that after I cut his hair, before he was buried, I would place my business cards by his head during the open casket. Maybe I could drum up some new business. I would place a little sign, HAIR BY DEBBIE. Now I was being the morbid one. Well, two could play at this game!

What about a casket cut fee? There should be a small fortune to pay for a service such as this! I would have to make a menu with services, the à la carte kind, and add a casket cut fee, since this was only an à la carte service, one-time fee. I would have to then take a deposit and the beneficiary of the will would have to pay the rest before I descended down the stairs to the basement for that final cut. Or maybe, I thought, I should charge in full now, to make sure I was compensated for the therapy I would be needing after the casket cut.

I told him, "No offense, but I cannot imagine touching you when you are dead." I would have to invest in a vacuum cutter. That way, I could put it on the setting I wanted, turn it on, and cut his hair without having to feel his cool stiffness. What about his eyebrows? I guessed they would be included, since I trimmed them now. I hoped he died with his eyes closed! Sometimes, I ran a little color through his "foreign" hair. I thought it would be too much maintenance. Once I had the color on, it had to process for a good twenty-five minutes. I remembered thinking, *What will I do while this is taking place?* Usually, I'd have lunch. I didn't think I would be having lunch! Then there was the shampoo. How would that be possible? That was not a one-man job. I mean, I was strong, but I couldn't lift a dead body, nor did I want to say I had lifted a dead body. Maybe I would just use the dark-colored hair spray they sold during Halloween season and spray that on. I would be in the room alone with him; no one would know but me. He reassured me I would have to do it the way I always did it if it was in his will. He always mentions his will and that it was in there, so I would be forced to do so. He said his grandson would come get me and take me to this basement where he would be, and there would only be one light on, swinging above his head, and I would be the only one in the room with him. The thought of that made me want to feed him vitamins.

He was also the client who was fortunate enough to have my underwear on his neck during my most embarrassing times behind the chair. In the new addition of his story of how I would be forced to cut his hair upon his death, he mentioned that he was updating his will, and I would have to cut his hair in the underwear that were on his neck. OK, that was well over eighteen years ago. If he thought I still had the same pair, he was mistaken.

"They should be framed somewhere," said the man who had haircut preparations in his will.

He had been a little under the weather, and I did not wish him unwell. Though, a little part of me wishes if he were to get sick and something bad were to happen, such as death—a long way down the road—that it would happen just after a haircut. Not four weeks out. If it was just after, my services would not be needed. I would be off the hook, and then I would feel so fortunate and would pay it forward, donating the money set aside for my services "down under" to my favorite charity. Or take up the therapy I had been saying I would need after such a discussion. You know the therapy would be about him. I would be lying on the couch talking about how he was going to make me cut his hair after he was gone, or if I had to cut it. It would be a weekly appointment based on a monthly discussion we always had about the casket cut.

Sometimes, he sits there with his eyes closed, relaxing. I tell him to open his eyes since he is freaking me out, making me think of the casket cut. He then crosses his hands on his chest. I think he is trying to prepare me, but there is no way I will ever do a casket cut!

THE MISCOMMUNICATION

Everyone's definition of an inch is different. If a lady client comes in and wants six inches off, I will first ask her to show me how much she wants off. She will hold up her hands and show me how much she thinks it is. I will show her my comb that has a ruler on it, and we will compare notes. If I took off the amount she said, it would surpass the amount she wanted by a few inches, and then I would have been a butcher.

Clients will say to me, "Just don't butcher it."

My response is usually as follows. "If I were going to be a butcher, I would be working behind a meat counter, wearing a white smock with my name tag on the left, over my heart." Or does it really matter which side your name tag is on? Are you planning on meeting people back in the cooler and have to have the proper name tag placement? If you're holding a cleaver, I bet there are not going to be many opportunities for meeting people. The same thing goes when they tell me not to chop it off. I am not a lumberjack with my ax; therefore, I will not be chopping anything off. It is important to let them know your occupation and that you do not moonlight.

You really must repeat back to the clients what you heard them say. Some clients will try to be all technical, but they really are unaware of the logistics of the hair terminology. For instance, they come in wanting highlights when they just applied a box color a week ago on their hair, coating every strand in dark brown or black, except for that one hard-to-reach patch they missed at the top of the occipital bone. They don't realize you work with a comb, not a magic wand. They want instant results, and they don't see what the big deal is. You could be drastic and give them what they want, but in the end, you don't want to jeopardize the health of their hair. A darker, even coating is much more elegant than orange fried cotton candy. I guess the best way to get that across is to collect such hair samples and then display them on a swatch, and when they are looking at the color book, wanting the impossible, you can point out the reality of the outcome. No one would pick that swatch choice.

Some clients will tell me to cut an inch off their bangs. If I cut an inch off their bangs, they will not only shrink up but they will have to walk around with their eyebrows raised for six weeks to close that forehead gap I was talking about. That would entail too much energy on their part. If I have a new client in, I will ask how he or she styles his or her hair, and how much time he or she spends. That way I can custom cut the client's hair, knowing he or she is not spending as much time styling as I am, and I will give the client a low maintenance style. I cannot cut the bangs short since it is my phobia. My mom used to cut my bangs, and she would tell me to sit still, and I would. Then she would tell me that she had to even them out. What did that mean? I was sitting like a statue. In all of my cutting days, I had never had to say those words. My bangs always ended up uneven and short with my mom's barbering. I brought in photos to share with clients as proof. "Don't let this happen to you" type of thing.

If clients want their bangs shorter, I will cut them shorter. If they ask for more off the third time, I want to make them sign something that releases me of any wrongdoings. A client came in one time on pain medication. She told me how she was seeing pink everywhere a few days earlier. She requested shorter bangs, and I had to ask her if she really thought she should make that call, since she was on meds and all and seeing pink clouds. I went back in and cut a few hairs, but mainly, I was just going through the motions. I didn't want her to sober up and wonder why they were so short and hate me.

I had a new walk-in client one afternoon. I was on my way out for the day, and she somehow made her way into my room, after making the rounds finding out everyone else was busy. I told her I would make an appointment for her for another day, but as I was doing so, she sat in my chair. I decided to just go ahead and deal with her then. She had just had a haircut a few days earlier but hated it. She wanted me to fix it. As I was cutting it, it was a little longer on one side, but other than that, it wasn't that off. She kept telling me she spent a lot of money on the cut and that she had the "style master" cut it, so she was shocked it was as bad as it was. She had a strong British accent. When I was finished, she stood to get a better look in the mirror. She pointed to a little spot by the right ear that she thought was longer, so I cut a little more off on that side. She pointed at it again and said it was still longer. I didn't think it was, and knew if I cut it, it would be shorter on that side now, so I faked cut it.

She looked again and said, "Perfect! It's just perfect!" I knew then that I was dealing with a nutbag. *Nutbag*: An odd, eccentric or insane person (not a scrotum).

She made another appointment a month out, but I had some dread brewing inside. As I went to work the next day, I asked a few ladies if they saw the British woman from the day before. A few of them had and also felt alarm toward her. I always try to give people the benefit of the doubt, and try to please them, because I am a true people pleaser, and that quality doesn't always work out for me. She came in for her second appointment, and she seemed fine. She did inspect the cut more than I was used to since I'd had clients for years, and they always knew it would be good. She liked to stand in the mirror and study it. I would tell her how lovely she looked and all of that, but after five minutes, her time was up. After the fourth booking, I called to remind her of her appointment the day before, and she acknowledged it, but then never showed. I made one more appointment for her, and she, once again, didn't show, so that was that. I never called her again, and one time I saw her at Fred Meyers, and I hid.

I got the feeling she wasn't happy with her life when she would share bits and pieces. She said (in her British accent) that her husband didn't like for her to wear shorts.

So she said, "I'm going to start doing what I like to do and wear them. In fact, I just bought three pairs." I thought that was all right. If she was happy wearing them, then she should; just don't stand me up.

A girl in beauty school was cutting a female client, when all of a sudden we heard screaming. The student was in tears; the client was yelling and jumping out of the chair, and we were all awaiting the outcome. Word finally made it to the dispensary that she had cut all of the woman's hair off. We finally found out that the client said to cut three inches off, and the student heard to leave three inches. Why the client wasn't watching the student in the first place was beyond me. It was a beauty school after all, and that was where we learned our lessons, from our mistakes and also from the mistakes of others. It makes you realize that miscommunication can ruin your look for months to come.

In beauty school, I had a male client in my chair who had not had a haircut in a very long time. Judging by his looks, he was stuck in the '70s. We consulted, and he wanted it shorter. He really didn't specify the length, so I would ask as I went to make sure. I asked him if he wanted it over his ears. He said that he did, so I cut it over his ear. I finished one side, and he was upset. He wanted it over his ears, meaning, to still cover his ears. Again, it was a beauty school, and we were still students, learning all of the new skills, so it was amazing to me how clients were not paying attention at these crucial times. Relaxing, reading a magazine is what you would do in a spa/salon setting around licensed hairdressers, not when you are paying a student in a beauty school three dollars. So now when I ask, I will ask them if they want it over their ears, meaning *up* over their ears, the ear exposed, all while pretending to be Vanna White, motioning with my hands. I have thought back about that over the years and how I really learned a lot that day by cutting that man's hair over his ears.

Thank goodness for beauty school. You learn how to communicate and really find out what the client has in mind. Otherwise, I would still be back home, cutting hair out in the yard with my twelve-dollar scissors, waiting for a reaction as to whether they liked it or not. Now, I am seasoned.

I like to say I am a seasoned hairdresser rather than an old hairdresser. It sounds much more professional. Clients ask if you have to take training every year to keep your license. I tell them there are no requirements for that. You keep your license as long as you pay your annual fee on time, and that is that.

"I do, however, like to stay current," I say. "That is why I'm seasoned."

THE THINGS YOU
SHOULD NOT SAY

One thing you should not do is guess what a client says. Once, I had a client in that I could not understand. I had to keep asking her to repeat what she had just said. After a while, I started guessing what I thought she said. I thought she said she was taking medication.

"No," she said, "I just got back from vacation." We didn't talk anymore after that, and I realized that I should no longer guess what a client is saying.

Then there are the things that come out wrong. I was walking a client out who just said he was going to have lunch.

I started to say, "Have a nice lunch, or a good day," but it came out, "Have a nice lay." He turned back around to me so fast and I quickly said, "Day!" A nearby stylist heard the whole conversation and started laughing, which only added to my embarrassment.

Also, you must be careful not to talk over the blow-dryer. This is how secrets get out. When you are under the dryer, you cannot hear as well, so you think that others cannot hear you. That is not the case. We can almost hear you better, since you are in that heated, noisy dome. It is the muffling what you are hearing, but projecting your voice out for everyone to hear, as if there is not enough room in there for the hot air to blow, plus your hot air.

I have clients who talk loud over the blow-dryer. I will look around to see if other stylists and clients are listening. You really cannot help yourself. I listen in next door all the time. It is funny; sometimes I will be listening to the conversations around me and not even notice that the radio has been on all along.

I am good at multitasking. I usually know what is going on a few stations away, who is coming in, leaving, and what clients are having for dinner. I do have a client who likes to cause a stir for fun.

Just out of the blue when I am cutting her hair, she will yell, "Ouch!" Then she will start laughing. She loves the reaction she gets, because everyone turns to see what is going on. I have to then redeem myself to them, letting them know I didn't just harm my client.

One thing that shouldn't be in your vocabulary is, "I am so happy you are my last client. I cannot wait to go home." That is only going to make your clients feel they are keeping you from something other than doing their hair. Now they are going to think you are not on your game and that you are rushing. No matter what, *never* make a client feel you would rather be doing anything else other than his or her hair. It is our job to make clients feel taken care of, pampered, and not left feeling guilty that they are holding you up. I used to work next to a stylist who would say such things. It made me feel bad for her clients. They also don't want to hear you are tired. The show must go on. You are on stage when you are doing hair. If you would rather be in the audience than performing, then take the day off, and let your understudy take over.

I had a young lady client in my chair. I was doing corrective color on her, so I was with her for some time. She kept hitting her teeth with her tongue piercing. The sound that it made was driving me crazy. I tried to ignore it, but she wasn't making it easy for me to do that, and I thought she wanted me to notice it. Believe me, everyone around her knew she had her tongue pierced. When I first heard the noise, I thought she was chewing on a Tic Tac. This lasted longer than that little mint, so I knew then that she indeed had a stud in her mouth. Did she need this much attention? Seemed as though you would be a little discreet if you got that type of piercing. Maybe she didn't realize what she was doing, sort of a nervous tic. Nothing grabs your attention like a studded tongue and a nervous tic. I had to excuse myself and go into the break room while her color was processing. I mentioned it to my fellow stylists. One guy asked me to ask her what else she had pierced. I wasn't sure I was ready for this.

I went back to check on her, and I said, "I see you have your tongue pierced." I was trying to act all calm, as if I came up with these questions all on my own. I didn't want her to think she was the topic of the roundtable in the break room, and that I was instructed to get her to open up. My first question was, "What else do you have pierced?" She told me she had her eyebrow pierced, which I had been trying not to comb and was aware of its whereabouts. Then she said her ears, her nipples, of course…"Oh, of course," I said, as if I was on board and my nipples were equipped with the same attire.

She continued with, "My navel and my hood." I went back to the break room and reported all her other piercings. I ended with the hood and asked what it was. When the answer was thrown my way, I said, "Of course." I guess I didn't know the real name to that part of my body. Now when I hear, "Let me check under your hood," I will know to slap my mechanic.

THE THINGS YOU
SHOULD NOT SEE

Clients like to show you things. Sometimes, it is just too much information. My eyes didn't need to see that. I guess they are close with you and feel the need to share.

I had a client in who started out calm. As the years progressed, she started going through a divorce, and I guess it was safe to say she grew a little wild. She started getting tattoos and piercing things. I am fine with that. I love seeing the tattoos since it is a form of art. I don't have any myself, but I can live vicariously through others with them. One day, she was talking about her new piercing. I asked her about it, and she said she would show it to me. I should have been suspicious when she got out her phone. She was getting the picture ready for viewing, making it bigger, and called my attention. I peered over her shoulder to see it is a double piercing…down below…in a place I did not have a need to see. I looked away from it so fast as if it were the sun, and it were burning my eyes. I couldn't believe she showed that to me. All I could say was,

"Oh, my eyes!" She was laughing. Now, when I think of her, that image comes into my mind. I don't want it there. I try to shake my head, as if it were an Etch A Sketch, wanting it to disappear, but that would be too easy.

EH EQUALS EAR HAIR

It happens to men as they get older. The dreaded ear hair. You almost hate to point it out—that the day has come, they have visible ear hair, and they are not walking out with it. Liquidation sale...it must go! If you have been cutting their hair forever, and you know this is the first time you have seen an ear hair, then you should point out what you are about to do. Trimming the ear hair can lead to many feelings. They may need consoling because they are probably feeling older upon their first hair there. They may go into denial and argue the fact that it is not really there, even though you are staring it in the face. Especially in the right light, there is no denying it is there. I have good ear hair eye sight, since I am used to looking for it, so I know what I am seeing. I am a trained professional. The fact is, once they starting having ear hair, it usually means they are losing it on their head. It seems the guys who have less hair on their heads have the most ear hair, so I always have a lot of extra work to do.

I have a client who likes to argue with me that I have never cut an ear hair from him. I remind him that I found one a few years ago. I can usually pinpoint the date and the day of the week, making it hard to argue with me, since I have presented my date memory on prior occasions. I did let it go the first time. I cut it in silence, not sharing with him his old man ears. Maybe this made him unaware it was there. He does wear glasses, and I thought he would hear the buzz from the clipper, but my bad. He was clueless of his ear hair. He must have thought I was just waving the clipper around, unaware I was cutting his first ear hair.

The second time I found an ear hair on him, I cut it and threatened to tape it to his card that was in the client card vault. Of course I would never do that. It's funny, just the thought of it, with him believing I would. I did save it one time while he went to the ATM to get the money he needed to pay me. Upon his return, I held the card containing his precious ear hair into the air and blew it to the floor, no longer holding it hostage until he returned with the cash.

The third time it happened, I looked for the ear hair when he first sat down. Jackpot! Now, I could just cut it and be done with it, but I couldn't do that. I had to point it out since he liked to argue about it. I told him the hair was back, and he denied it, so I pulled on it.

He finally said, "Ouch!"

I said, "See, you do have an EH." He even knew that EH stood for *ear hair*. He had to admit to it since the tug on the hair was starting to hurt. He was bending his head as I gripped the hair with a look of defeat. I felt a little victorious and tried not to fully extend my smile, as if to say I had won. I would keep an eye on it. It had a pattern now of showing up about every third haircut. I had to admit, it was a little scary that I knew the growth rate of ear hair.

I also have two other male clients who each have a lone hair that grows out of the backside of the ear. Near the end of the appointment, as I am dusting them off, I hunt for it, and make sure I got it.

109

Usually when you first find one and cut it, they ask to see it. I have done some fast thinking, and I picked up a random cut hair that may have been near—perhaps one from the head that had collected on the shoulder of the cape that was longer than the actual ear hair—and showed it to them. They say, "I can't believe it would be that long without me noticing!" I then have to laugh and reveal my brattiness, that the hair I just showed them was from their head. It never gets tiring trying to fool them.

Another client has a lot of ear hair that I always get rid of. He knows when it is time.

As I get the clippers out and start to go in, he always says, "Those are long. You forgot to cut them last time."

Right! I never forget to cut them, and as I am cutting them, I say, "I am not forgetting to cut these." They are long. I could practice some braiding right now. He likes to blame me for some reason on their growth rate, as if I have applied some secret hair growth serum on them when he wasn't looking. As I am cutting them, I have to really press on the backside of the ear to make it plush so I can really get in there and get all of the hair hiding in their crannies. No, I would never forget! What would that mean for me? It would mean he would make a special trip in one day while he was driving, tugging on his ear hair, thinking of how I forget to cut them, and now I owed him, somehow, a free ear hair trim. Well, no thank you.

An occasional woman has had an ear hair. What do I do? Do I tell her? Do I offer to tweeze it? For some reason, if it is a woman, I would not swipe it with a clipper. If it's a guy, I'm swiping all over. With women, a clipper seems to be too delicate of a subject to approach, making them question a random growth of ear hair. It doesn't matter if there is just one; there may as well be ten. It's all the same. Ear hair…it's not for women.

A hair, no matter the location, can easily and discreetly be removed quickly with tweezers, no questions asked. Except, in an indoor voice after looking around to make sure the coast is clear, out of earshot of others to hear, "Do you want me to tweeze that?" A woman's hair is a secret and deserves to have anonymity. A man's, no big deal. We all accept that men are hairy.

I had a guy come in whom I had not seen in nearly three years. His hair was long and out of shape, and he did admit that he'd had a few hair affairs along the way. At first glance, I knew he had, but he felt the need to come clean. I jokingly said that I had not seen him for so long and wondered if he had any ear hair yet. He said he didn't, but toward the end, I zoned in on one and had to point it out.

All he said was, "Get it!" Some guys are embarrassed by their first ear hair, but I am used to it and see it all day long, so it is nothing new to me. The thing I am not used to is the nose hair. I draw the line there. They can "get that" on their own time in the privacy of their own bathroom mirror.

One client asked me if I cut nose hair. I had to stop cutting to look at him and tell him, "I do not cut nose hair." He said, "Oh, I thought you did." I said, "I have never cut nose hair." He looked up in the air, as if he was recalling a time when I cut his nose hair. I added, "I draw the line at nose hair." Really? I had to declare that aloud? Why would clients want me to take my clipper to that area? They need to go to the store and purchase a nose hair trimmer and do it for themselves in the privacy of their own facilities. You just cannot pay me enough to have to do that. It will never be on my list of services. Not even if it were a fancier name, such as nostril locks. It's never going to happen. I have trimmed the top of the mustache, before it starts to mingle with the unconfined nose hair. Nose hair and the upper mustache hair should not intertwine. There should be a visible line between them.

I had a client in who had the biggest patch of unkempt nose hair. I tried not to stare at it, as in disbelief of the abundance. It looked like Barbie's armpit hair, if she were European, and I wondered how it went unnoticed.

I do cut eyebrows. It ties into the haircut, making guys look less *professorish* and more tamed.

One of my clients called it "his brow," and as I trimmed them with my clippers, he said, "Wow! That actually made the lights dim," even though my clippers were cordless. His eyebrows have turned white, so I put a little color on them, tying them into the color on his head. I have had women who have had a long stray eyebrow hair, and I used to be shy about not pointing it out, but I figured I would want to know, so I would get it for them.

One lady responded after I told her of her long eyebrow hair, "I do? It's like a curtain up there. I had no idea."

I recently had a client who had a very long ear hair. At first when I saw it, I thought it was a fallen hair that had collected into his ear. As I took the towel to dust around his ears, freeing all of the hair that may have fallen in, I noticed it didn't budge. I pulled on it and found it was attached. I decided to get my tweezers out, which was a very serious matter.

I told him, "This is a very serious matter. I am getting my tweezers out." As I grasped the hair in my tweezers grip, I gave a yank, and it came up clean. I was shocked that I missed it since it was so apparently chilling there, as if it had no place to go. I tried again and missed. OK, now I was serious, I announced again, and I focused on the hair and gave it another tug, and with the tension, I felt I had succeeded. I looked at the tweezers, and in its clutches, there was an inch-long hair. I had no idea how this inch-long hair could have been hiding in the ear. Hair grows a half inch a month. That hair had been there for two haircuts. I didn't know how I could have missed it.

I asked him, "How did you not feel that hair? Was it not all itchy in there, as if a cockroach or something was nesting in there?" He said he never felt a thing.

The thing that baffled me was when I saw it in his ear, it looked small. As I looked at it in its entirety, it had to have been rooted way back into his ear canal. That was a first, and it was a mystery. I didn't have a clue as to how a hair could grow deep in the dark depths of the ear canal. It's like the forest floor that had never seen the sun. Yet, there it was, tucked into a coiled ball, the tip exposed for my pulling. And I pulled. I was not shy. The client was in a month later, and he said he thought he had another hair growing in the other ear. I took a gander, and he was right. I got my tweezers out, gave it a quick, easier-to-pull-this-time tug, and he didn't even flinch. I asked if he felt that.

He said, "Not like the last time. I felt a pull on my ear drum on the other one." Looks like now I was on EH watch.

Whenever I get my tweezers out, to pull a stray hair, I tell clients to "Ask me about my one buck pluck." I tell them, it is a buck a pluck, and how I am going to have buttons made with that slogan, since my clientele is getting hairier.

THE CHILD'S HAIRCUT

I have started off with so many clients who were children. You dread the appointment, the screaming, the wiggling; you even sweat a little. They are afraid of the word "haircut," because they hear "cut," and it makes them think it will hurt. I have learned to change my wording to, "Let's go fix your hair." It sounds better, and once they get to my station and see the candy bowl, they are putty in my hands, for a few seconds. Once they start in on their squirming, I tell them to keep their eye on the bowl. I reassure them that if they sit still, I will let them have more than one piece of candy. It does help. If it doesn't, I let them sample a piece and then put the bowl away, so they know what they are going to miss out on. Sometimes, it works. I will do little tricks to take their minds off the haircut. I used to have a Ping-Pong ball that had an eyeball painted on it. I would hold it up into the flow of my blow-dryer, and it would just dance above the stream of invisible air, making them think I was pretty cool. Cool enough to keep them still for a little bit.

Eventually they get older, sit better, and you can really enjoy their visits. I had a little boy client who I dreaded. I would see his name on my schedule and try to come up with a way to get out of it. He would only be rescheduled, so I thought it best to just get it out of the way. He would rip the cape off, throw it on the floor, jump down and run. I had to go in search of him so that I would not leave him unevenly sheared. One time, I went out to the waiting area where his mom was sitting. I asked her if she had seen him. Great! I had lost her child. I went back to my station and asked my fellow stylists if they had seen him.

I said, "He is driving me crazy!" He came out of hiding and mimicked me, with his hand on his hip as I had done.

"He's driving me crazy!" he said. I told him to get back in my chair, after I informed his mother of his whereabouts.

He went through a faze where he wanted to be like Alfalfa. Although, he was blond, unlike Alfalfa, but that didn't matter. I would gel his hair, part it down the center, and make his back cowlick stand on end. He would walk out of the salon so proud. He grew older and turned into a nice young teen, and I enjoyed his visits in my chair. We had nice conversations, and I looked forward to seeing him, to catch up. We liked to reminisce about all of his bratty times in my chair. It was always good for a laugh, and I felt very blessed to have seen him grow up.

I have another young man who I have cut since he was in fourth grade. He came in one last time before going off to college. I told myself I was not going to have any tears when we said our good-byes. He gave me a big hug, and I told him he should leave before I started to cry. I was sort of joking, but then I did start to cry. Turned out I had empty chair syndrome.

I have a girl client who has come to me since her first haircut. I tried to cut her hair while her dad filmed the whole thing. Of course, she wouldn't stay still since she didn't really know about the sitting etiquette and didn't really care about the outcome of her hair. She was just enjoying the excitement of it all. It got to the point where she wanted out of my chair. I still had a few snips to make, since I couldn't let it go and wanted it to be perfect. As she was crawling around, I was crawling around behind her, trying to finish. Finally, I told her dad I was finished.

He said, "Are you sure you want to be finished?" Well, I was sure...I wanted to be finished before I started practically doing lunges and nearly the splits. I was getting a better workout than I would in a yoga class. Throughout the years, she learned to sit still, and I got to do her monumental hairdos, such as eighth-grade graduation, high school prom, and senior pictures. Now, she has graduated from high school, and I see her when she comes home from college. I have asked her dad from time to time if I could watch the video of the first haircut, twenty-three years ago. He brought in a copy for me a few Christmases ago, so I could watch it. I had to laugh at my attire. I couldn't believe I used to think I was fashionable with a floral print dress and white nylons, but the cutting dedication, crawling on the floor behind her to finish, impressed me.

One little boy was due in for his haircut. I saw his mom carrying him, asleep. I was thinking this could be good or very bad. Maybe he would be subdued. She sat him in the chair, and the minute he saw where he was, he started screaming and crying. I couldn't work on a loud client and let it interrupt all of the other relaxed patrons, so we had to reschedule. That was when I was not excited to see kids on my schedule: if it takes two appointments to get the job done and you only get paid for the one.

Another little boy was screaming so loud that I did have to escort him out in his mother's arms. When we were outside, she asked if I could just cut it outside. I decided to give it a try since he would just have to schedule another appointment spot. She stood there holding him while I worked as fast as I could. Clients going in to the salon got a kick out of it and wondered if they too could get their hair done outside.

I have a client whom I cut when he was seven years old. He is now thirty-five. He lives out of town, but when he comes to visit his parents, he comes in to see me. The last time I cut his hair, after the cut, I overheard him talking to his mom.

He said, "There is just no one who can cut my hair like Debbie." I was so touched by that. It sort of puffed up my pride and my head got a little heavy.

The little clients I have now are good. They sit still and like to come in. They keep their eyes on the candy bowl, and sometimes, when I make homemade cookies, they really have something to look forward to. Such an indulgence to look for when it is over. Two of my clients actually sit better than their dad. They laugh when I tell them this.

One of my clients started coming to me when she was twelve. She is now thirty-six, married, and has two kids. I was so happy to do her wedding hair. There we were, in the middle of the curling and pinning, and I started to tell her what a beautiful bride she was going to make, and how happy I was to have seen her grow into a beautiful lady, getting to do her hair for her special day. I started getting misty eyed and had to excuse myself and wipe my tears. It was a little embarrassing, and when it happened a second time, I decided not to hide the fact that I sometimes got a little emotional.

It was hard on the days I would get four kids in a row, all under the age of five. My nerves would be shot, and when you are a single, working mother, you go to work to be with adults and don't want to be around kids all day who will not sit still, since you get to do that at home. I used to joke about how I would go to work to relax, so the kids haircuts had to stop. I started refusing new kid clients. One day, a lady called and tried to get in with her child. I told her I was no longer taking new kid clients.

She pulled the 'ole name dropping trick, saying, "So and so referred her."

I said in return, "So." I knew I needed a break.

I was in the break room one day, with only a few minutes for my lunch, and another stylist came in and asked me if I would wipe her client's child's butt! I looked at her between my bites and wondered if I heard her correctly. She repeated the statement again. I asked her why she needed me to do this task.

"Well, I'm busy, my client is under the dryer, and you are a mom."

"And how old is the child?" I asked. She was four. I inquired more, asking if the mother was OK with a stranger wiping her child's butt. Apparently, she was and didn't want to do it. She wanted to stay under the dryer while her hair color was processing and continue reading magazines. I too was a mother and would love to choose that option, but you cannot go around letting strangers wipe your child's butt. I told her I only had a minute to finish my sandwich, and I did not come to work today to wipe a butt! That was the end of that.

THE DEB SCRUB

I really like to pamper my clients at the shampoo bowl. They love the special treatment they get. It is their time to relax, rejoice, and tune out the worries of their day. I try to make them leave their stress at the bowl, because once they are all minty and ready for the haircut, they are like putty in my hands. The shampooing techniques I use to gain their trust; the neck massage leaves them easy going.

You can tell the ones who really love it. They get to the bowl and really settle in, ready to be pampered. I will spend a sufficient amount of time massaging the neck. It is best if a client lets me pick up his or her head, otherwise, when I am rinsing, I will give him or her a bath. One client popped up the minute I was in lather mode. I tried to gently push his head back down, but he had the strongest neck muscles. I then had to tell him the importance of bowl contact. If the client didn't keep contact with the bowl, while I was rinsing, water would shoot down his back, then I would have to spend extra time blow-drying his shirt. Although, one size does not fit all, and some clients cannot mold to the bowl, so they get wet.

You know the clients who are not ready to be done at the bowl. You massage the neck and try to get them to relax, but they will just not put their head back down in the bowl, as if they are holding it up to get more. This bargaining tool is nice to use. If they are late for their appointment, you can tell them you will not have time for a lengthy shampoo, and it will make them be on time.

I always wish we could have a no talking zone in the shampoo room. It should be a quiet sanctuary where our clients can de-stress and take a moment for themselves. Sort of like during a massage. There is not a lot of talking going on in there. It's hard when I am trying to relax my client, and another person is carrying on, enough for my client to open his or her eyes and give me that look. I try to look at the person who is unaware of their volume, but they do not seem to get it.

I have said aloud, "Hey, this is a no talking, quiet zone…" Still, the person doesn't get it and just keeps blathering on. I then want to say, in a voice that can be heard, "Don't blather…lather!"

I now work in a studio all to myself, so I can control the shampoo setting. I have soft lighting for when I turn the overhead lighting off, so it isn't so bright in their eyes, and they cannot look up my nose. I will adjust my music more softly, and I try not to talk, unless they do. My clients love it, but it does make it harder when I have to turn the lights back on. Also, the nice thing about having your own personal bowl, is that it is always how you left it. It was always so embarrassing when you would take your client to a shampoo bowl after sloppy coworkers who left suds and hairballs all over it, and occasionally, hair color would get on your clothes from them, since they forgot their mothers didn't work there.

I really get a workout while shampooing. I put a lot of muscle into it. I tell my clients that it cuts my workout time down, so please don't be late. I would hate to have to join a gym. I worked next to a girl who would really get into the back combing while wearing sleeveless tops. One day, while she was really working on her teasing technique, she looked at me from under her arm and shook it as we watch a little bit of flab from under her arm swing back and forth. I knew then she didn't spend enough time shampooing.

Another time, she decided to grow her underarm hair out and quit shaving. I still to this day haven't a clue for her decision. She was not French. In fact, she was Italian and always complained how hairy she was. I have never in my life had an underarm hair goal and haven't known any other woman who has. There she was, in the back-combing position, picking and spraying while finishing a do. I watched her spray the hairspray in a continual motion from her client, to under her armpit, while she fluffed her armpit hair with the comb. She knew I was watching and wanted to amuse me. She was fun to work next to, and we used to laugh a lot with the clients. We had a discussion around the break room table one day about trimming your hair "down there." She said it had never occurred to her to trim it.

She said, "I'm Italian! I could probably go down a pant size if I trimmed it!" After that, I referred to her as Fluffy.

I have a couple of clients who do not like the shampoo. One client doesn't know why I would waste my time at the shampoo bowl. She wants me to just lather, rinse, condition, and go.

Another client, after five years of the pampering shampoo told me, "That is about enough scrubbing back there!" I thought she was saying, "I will give you an hour to stop that." I have heard that before, from several clients. Most clients say to just skip the haircut and continue the shampoo. This client was getting testy, so I asked her if she wanted me to stop massaging. She did! She said she didn't like it. So for five years, she let me hold her hostage at the bowl and do what I thought was a luxury? Why not just say so in the beginning, and I could also save my hard-working upper body strength for a client who would appreciate it?

Another client has never had me shampoo his hair. I just spray him down with the water bottle. He doesn't know what he is missing. It makes me wonder if he had ever had a real shampoo and just had a bad experience, or if he had never made that transformation from the kids' cut to the real deal. When little kids are in, I usually just get their hair wet with a spray bottle, since they have a hard time fitting in the shampoo bowl, partially due to their size and for the fact they are usually ready to bolt from the chair the moment they hear the water turn on and whirl under their head. This man's wife loves the shampoo. She tells me she will take his, along with hers, so it is extended.

I have had an occasional client who had vertigo and cannot lean back into the shampoo bowl. It is hard to really offer my services when they are face down in the bowl since there is nothing that supports their head, so I feel they are missing out on the pampering and are usually ready for it to be over. I know it is best for them, so I am accommodating. I just want them to be comfortable, which is providing a great service after all, the custom-made kind.

I have an older lady who cannot lean back far enough to reach the bowl. She leans back, and there is about six inches between her neckline and the lip of the bowl. There is no way you are going to turn the water on. It doesn't take a rocket scientist to know you are not going to keep them dry. I found a little plastic rinsing cape that goes around the neck. I have her hold onto the straps of it, and it stays snug against her neck. I funnel the rest of the water into the bowl, and the water runs down it, into the bowl, sort of like a water slide, minus the fun music. The little strip of plastic keeps her bone dry, except for one time when the plastic wasn't all the way in the bowl, and after it collected enough water, it gave way onto the floor. That was not a good deal all together. Then you not only have to be a janitor but a launderer as well.

A guy client I've had for twenty-four years always goes ahead of me and sits in the shampoo chair, saying it's time for his bath. He is already in the reclined position by the time I grab my towel and meet him there. I struggle to get him to sit up enough to slip my towel under his neck. While I am rinsing, he always says that the water just ran all the way down his back. I reassure him it didn't.

Again, with another rinsing session, he says, "That one made it all the way down to my butt!" Then he will take a drop of the water, maybe from a splash that landed on his forehead, and flick it, as to make a point. When he sits up to go back to my station, I make sure to point out to him that he is completely dry.

A new guy client was in, and after the shampoo, I had him sit up so I could towel dry his hair, so he would not have to drip back to my station. The towel I placed around his neck started to fall to the floor. I caught it in time, but ended up grabbing his bottom! I assure you, it was accidental. The next time he came in, he tried to get the towel to fall, in hopes to get another bottom grab out of me. Another client always takes the towel, spins it around, and tries to snap me with it, or some of the other stylists, which of course is frowned upon in a professional environment, and it dawned on me this was what horseplay was. As a child, when I would go to the swimming pool in the summer, I read the list of pool rules that were posted, and one of the rules was no horseplay. I thought that was funny, since we were not animals. At least, I will speak for myself, but I am finding out that some clients can be so frisky after the shampoo. I wonder sometimes what is going on and why there is movement when they are sitting there with their hands under the cape and there is a weird motion going on.

I want to say, "Put your hands where I can see them." One time, I had a guy in who was a heavy breather. I was getting worried since he was so focused with something under the cape. It wanted to say, "What are you doing? Knitting under there?" If I pull the cape away, there better be a potholder or the beginnings of a scarf!"

On occasion, the hose from the shampoo bowl has gotten away, and I would try to turn the water off as quickly as it registers I had lost control. I hope I had not soaked my client and everyone around the vicinity. Another stylist in the bowl behind me lost control of the hose one time, and it soaked me, saturating through my pants. I had water dripping down my legs. The next time, we were at the bowls together, and I was behind him, I threatened a pay back, but never had the misfortune.

He said, "Go ahead. I've got my rubber underwear on."

Another male stylist I worked with taught himself to shampoo from the right side of the bowl, opposite from the rest of us. It could get a little crowded when you were shampooing at the same time. I noticed when he cut, he used his right hand. So I had to ask him if he was right or left handed. He told me he was right handed but liked to shampoo on the other side so he could be cheek to cheek with the girls. When I had been shampooing behind him, he would stick his bottom and bump mine, as if we were playing tag. Sometimes I would do the same, and then he would do it again, and then I thought he had this all figured out, rubbing bottoms with the girls.

In another salon where I was working, the bowls were out from the wall, so you could stand behind the bowl. It was so much better for my back. I learned new ways to massage, and different angles. It was working for me, as I was having less pain in my shoulders at the end of the day. The faucet handle was different, however, and it was a lever. I was used to knobs. My sleeve got caught on it one time, and as I lifted my arm, I lifted the lever, turning the water on, and it shot over my client. It was such a sudden shock for both of us. I found it best to not wear big sleeves around the shampoo bowls, for fear of repeated occurrences. I never thought there would be a dress code for different styles of shampoo bowls.

CAN'T HANDLE THE PRESSURE

I have a client who doesn't have as much hair. I still go through all of the motions that I go through with those more follically fortunate. However, when I am rinsing the shampoo, if I turn the water pressure up too high, the moment it hits his bald head, it ricochets off his head onto me and gets me wet. It can be a problem if I am wearing something that is dry clean only. I must remember to always start with a low flow of water. This way, I will not have to adjust it and make him wonder why I am messing around so much with the water, which makes me wonder if he automatically assumes we have to worst water pressure in our salon.

Beside the Bowl Again
I never thought I would be a bowl snob, but as it turns out, I am. I used the same type of shampoo bowl for most of my career. The ones that only allow me to stand beside my client as I pamper them, freezing me into a partial right bend, with my left elbow in the air. Then I moved to a new salon and started using the bowls that actually allowed you to stand behind the bowl. It

makes sense. It is ergonomically correct. No more bending and twisting. No more back and shoulder pain. It took a while to get used to the new style of bowls, and I am not sure all of the clients were crazy about them. As I watched others shampooing their clients, the clients would make faces as they were getting soaked. The key to keeping the client dry was by cupping. Cupping is when you use your hand as a shield around the hairline while you are rinsing. This barrier will take on the splashes so your client's face doesn't have to. Some of the older ladies who wear more makeup appreciate this technique. That way, when you are done, they do not have that white line between the edge of the face and the hairline, where the makeup used to be before you savagely splashed it off. Also, clients with the painted-on eyebrows will benefit as well, as long as you are careful not to grace them with the towel as you are drying.

As I moved once again to another salon, the deal breaker for me was the correct shampoo bowls. It was nice to be able to get behind the bowl, and I have learned a few new scrubbing techniques. I point them out to the clients and they give me their feedback. It is usually good, as long as I keep them dry. Also, as I am shampooing behind the bowl, I stand wider than shoulder length and bend my knees, so I get a good squat exercise at the same time. This way, my body is lower, and I do not have to lean forward and strain my back. Win-win situation.

As a stylist, you spend so much time at the bowl; you have to envision yourself there, lathering, rinsing, repeating. It is not the most important thing, but it is part of the experience I give to my clients, so it is important enough. Plus, I don't want to strain my back. I get up earlier in the morning to stretch.

I tell my clients that I say to myself, "I am going to be doing hair today, so I need to stretch." I want to remain limber for this job. I walked into a new salon and felt like I was home. It has been so long since I have felt like that. The bowls are not the kind I prefer, but they will do since I love everything else. At least they are higher, so I don't have to bend as much.

I was in a salon for nearly fifteen years when it sold. Some of us ventured out and opened a new salon. I helped with putting it together, the painting, buying dishes for the break room, all sorts of ways to help with getting it open on time. We worked with the same receptionist for all of those years, and I was so happy she was going to be once again at the front desk. As time went on, she told us she wasn't getting paid what she was promised, so she ended up quitting. We were all upset by this, so a meeting was held to discuss such topics. I mentioned that our rent went up quite a bit from what we were told it would be, and we were led to believe the receptionist would be fairly compensated. Other stylists spoke their minds more than I had done. When I went to work the next day, I was asked to talk to the owner. I told her I only had ten minutes to eat lunch and my client was due in, so we would have to talk later. She really wanted to talk to me that minute. She told me I was fired! I was given a two-week notice slip. The worst part about it was my client was in and there I was, crying uncontrollably. I couldn't believe she did that right before my client was due to arrive. Just one of the many unprofessional things she did, but in the long run, it ended up being for the best. She fired another stylist as well.

When asked the reason behind the termination, I was told, "Since the receptionist left and was causing problems, you have to go too. You are the posse." I was? I had barely even ridden a horse! How could you be part of a posse and not even know it? I'm pretty sure you choose this alliance, and if I was going to truly be in a posse, I was so going to own it!

I really don't like moving around to different salons. I am not a salon hopper, but it is important to find the right fit. It is not fun to work in a place you are so unhappy in and cannot wait to go home to have a cry. I worked shortly in a salon that made me do just that. It was one big room that contained four chairs, lined up in a tight row, the waiting room and the shampoo bowls all in one room. It was very loud in there, as it was a stone building, with tile everywhere, nothing to soften the noise. There was no relaxing, no peace. If one of the other stylists was talking, you could not hear your client, or have private conversations. The other workers there, including the owner, would help themselves to my stuff, turning on my flat iron, or using my blow-dryer. I felt so invaded. The shampoo bowls were the only thing I liked, but that was not enough to make me stay and keep working in such horrible conditions. When my clients were voicing how unhappy they were there, I knew it was time to find a new place to work. It got worse after I gave my months' notice. I was treated as an outsider. I had a stack of fliers for my clients, with the information about the new location I was moving to. I came in one morning and my fliers were gone from my top drawer.

I told the owner about the missing fliers, and she said, "You think I took them?"

I said, "I never said that."

"Well, I don't want any of your clients. They're all old," she replied. There was nothing to do but walk away from her. She was totally disrespectful, and not worth any more of my time. Later, she came up to me to say that she knew who took my fliers, that it was caught on video. She always claimed she had cameras in the room, so she always knew what was going on, but she never let me see the footage.

Everyone else who worked there said they would bet it was the owner who took them, since she liked to stir up drama. She went through so many receptionists in the eight months I lasted there, due to her disrespectful authority. I was so happy to get out of that salon.

So now, I am in my studio with just my clients. It is peaceful, and we can talk if we want. We are not overpowered with clueless, loud stylists, so there is real pampering going on, which not only keeps my client in a relaxed state but it makes me feel relaxed. I just settle in at the bowl, and sometimes I sing a little song to my clients, "Beside the bowl again..."

My chair is next to my shampoo bowl, so all I have to do is turn my clients around and lower them down for the shampoo. Once they come in, they don't have to get up at all, unless they want to sit on my couch while their color is processing to use the foot massager and read a magazine. Sometimes a client will reach to turn on the shampoo bowl water, thinking he or she needs to rinse his or her hands or glasses, and the hose will rise and spray the client, or the hose will get away and spray the room.

As the client is reaching for the nozzle, I quickly scream, "No," and the person will stop, looking all childish like, as if he or she is being scolded, but I don't want him or her to get soaked. I say, "Look where the hose is aimed. Right at you." I do have another sink in the room for your washing needs. I was cleaning the bowl one day as my client was sitting on the couch across the studio, writing her check. I bumped the nozzle, and the water turned on and shot water all over her legs and feet.

We both screamed and she said, "I thought you were purposely doing that, since it is hot outside." Right. She had known me for thirty years, and knew how anal I was. Did she really think I wanted to mop up the studio?

COMB-OVER REMOVAL

There should be a special for a service such as this. In fact, if a guy were to sit in my chair with a comb-over, I would gladly remove it for free. For it is my civic duty. Maybe there should be one day of the month where they can all come in to get this taken care of.

Why is this look popular with the guys who are follically challenged? Who do they think they are kidding? We all know that under those long scraps is a bald head. You are not fooling anyone. It has to be more work placing it, combing it, and cementing it down. Why not just get it removed and be free? You know it is out of control when it starts wearing you, as if it has taken over your entire being, and there is no taming the beast, unless you see a professional who can help remove the burden. No one is going to voluntarily give it up. This is something they have to be talked into doing, like an intervention needs to take place with all of the comb-over guys' friends and families, immediately followed by a car ride to the hair salon.

There are two ways guys who wear the comb-over will comb this style into place. One way is the guy who actually uses the hand mirror to see the back, and knows how to sculpt it down into place. He combs it with special thought and care, placing each strand carefully, as to cover the bare or thinning spots. It is like solving a puzzle. He then sprays the heck out of it and avoids going outside on windy days. The second way is the guy who gives it a once over every now and again, who carries his comb in his pocket and combs it by feel. He doesn't care about the loose hairs that have not made it over to the other side and are dangling free, longer than the actual hairline, as if they are trying to escape and know they don't belong, begging to be noticed so they can be free of this style that is not fooling anyone. This guy usually uses the stylings of Brylcreem, believing the greasy substance will not only hold his hair in place, but make it seem thicker, because in his mind, it hasn't let him down since 1942.

I have a couple of clients who have the donut cut. It is refreshing to know they are accepting that bald is beautiful. One of the men started coming to me twenty-four years ago. I didn't think I would cut his hair for very long, since he seemed to be losing it, but he is still with me. He has the same amount of hair, and turns out, he likes being groomed and pampered. Besides, it would be boring if everyone had the same amount of hair.

I once had a client in from out of town. He was from a small town, and he had a comb-over. The minute I saw him, I tried to talk him out of it, but his wife wanted him to keep it. I could not believe I was cutting a comb-over. It just felt wrong.

When I was done with his hair, his wife was next in my chair. Meanwhile, her husband was outside in the wind, and his hair was blowing all around, as if he were in a convertible and the top was down. It was such a sight that I pointed him out to his wife.

I said, "Look at him out there. His hair is blowing all around. I wish he would let me cut his comb-over off. It would look much better." It turned out that she was the one who made him keep it. Every morning she combed and sprayed it into place. He hated it and wanted it gone. I talked her into letting me cut it off. When

I told him of our plan, he sat right down in my chair. He was so happy to have that thing gone. He said he felt so light and free.

About eight months later, he came back into town and found me. The stylist back home would not cut it off, since his wife thought he looked younger with more hair. Sometimes, hair can be a security blanket, but the spouse should get her own. After I moved from that salon, I never saw him again since I didn't have his address to notify him of my whereabouts. I think of him when I see a comb-over and wonder if he is still light and free.

The worst comb-over I ever saw was one that started at the nape of the neck and was combed upward, and over, settling on the forehead as straight across bangs — like Moe from the Three Stooges. I was behind him in line at the supermarket. As I awaited my turn, I studied it and wondered how people came up with such a bad idea. When they are first losing their hair, do they part it differently and then never get any cut off the long piece, until that piece is so long it becomes their security blanket and they cannot part with it? If you have to wrap it around your head a couple of times, you are asking for attention. It is a mystery you cannot solve, until you start to lose your hair.

How about the balding guys who have a few sparse threads of hair on the top of their head and then a long ponytail? This is just as bad as a comb-over. This showcases they know they are going bald, so they are going to grow it and keep as much as they can for as long as they can. This gives them many options—there is enough hair there in the back to make a hair turban.

My uncle had the long-ponytail balding-combination hairdo that he tied back. It would be worse if it were down, unless he was getting paid to smash watermelons, like the comedic stylings of Gallagher. One day, he let me cut it off. I cut it off above the rubber band, and he took it home as his hair trophy, probably because he would never in his life have that amount of hair again. He asked me not to tell anyone about his change. The next family gathering was for my grandma's eightieth birthday celebration. He came strolling in with a hat on, and when he turned around, his ponytail cascaded down his back. I knew it was gone, but he didn't want anyone to know. He had it clipped into his hat, and when it was time for my grandma to open gifts, his card was sitting on top of the pile. As soon as my grandma opened it, his ponytail fell out in her lap. The look on her face was priceless. He then removed his hat, revealing the short, nice haircut I had given him, the appropriate kind for thinning hair, and just stood there with a grin.

I decided to take a bow, and said, "My work here is done."

PRODUCT KNOWLEDGE

As a young girl, I bought into the idea of products. I would see an ad for a beauty regimen and want it. I was convinced of the greatness they provided in a single application, or by using the product, my life would change for the better. The only thing was, I lived in a small town, and you had to travel to get such items.

The day I saw No More Tangles stocked on the shelf, I zoned right in on it. The feel of the actual product in my hand—and the way I dreamed in my head that I would convince my mom how I *needed* it—consumed me. I held onto it, halfway wanting my mom to see it in my hand—that way it might dawn on her how I needed it, and then I would not have to find a way to ask for it—and halfway hiding it until I summoned the courage to convince her I had tangles and would actually die of exhaustion from combing out my hair without this product. I could have discreetly placed it in the shopping cart, under the loaf of Franz bread, then carried the groceries in and quickly hidden it, but she always checked the receipt, and I didn't want to seem untruthful. Even at the age of ten, I had integrity.

I guess I was not a good enough actor, because she didn't buy that I could not live without it, or rather, my hair would have to remain a knotted mess for the rest of my childhood, whichever came first. The truth was, I really didn't have a lot of tangles, and my hair was long. I just liked the idea of having a product of my own. Nonetheless, the girl on the bottle seemed about my age, with long blonde hair, like me, and I felt connected to her somehow. I pretended it was me on the label. It was the first product that I had seen from an ad that had actually been stocked on the shelves of my local grocery store. There were three bottles in stock. It was located on the middle shelf. I could not go into the store without at least going over to it, feeling it in my hand and reading up on it. It occurred to me I should hide a bottle incase three other girls had a tangle urgency and my mom came to her senses to buy it for me. To me, it was a big deal.

Those shampoo commercials, the ones with the excited girls in the shower, with the strawberry scented lather. Who were those women? I didn't have a clue, but I wanted to use what they were using. I thought I would feel aroused, plus, have the shiniest hair in town. Still, my mom was not buying it, and I feared I must go earn my own money to buy my own products. Was it because she feared I would go around, flipping my hair all around?

I also wanted No More Tears. Once again, I told my mom that if she were to buy No More Tears for me, even though it was for babies, my eyes would no longer have to suffer from all of the shampooing I had to do to keep my hair silky since she would not buy the No More Tangles. I remembered a period there where my mom stopped taking me along with her to the store. Now, I know why.

I was going to the eighth grade prom with the love of my life. I was a year younger than he was, and I already knew we would sail off into the sunset. Even more so if I used Gee Your Hair Smells Terrific Shampoo and Conditioner. This was a big selling grocery store brand product, with commercials that made you dream of purchasing, so you would be noticed for your lovely aroma. I just knew that if I were to slow dance with him after using that product, he would be mine. Somehow, I got my hands on some and was all ready for the dance. A slow song started to play, and it was my big moment. I rested my head on his shoulder, and waited. He never said a thing about my terrific smelling hair. I really thought he would sniff me and say, "Gee, your hair smells terrific." I thought I was going to have a moment right there in the Lincoln Junior High School gym with the love of my life. I could even smell my hair. It did smell pretty terrific. I decided he was missing out and that there would be no sunset.

Whenever I would hear of a new product that seemed so ridiculous, yet it worked, I would say, "What next? Debbie McRoberts hairspray?" I thought this was so funny, because it was so out there, as if I would have my own hairspray in my hand.

How about the Tickle? Now that was a phallic deodorant. I felt strange even grabbing it off the shelf and putting it in my shopping basket, as if I were being judged. I never knew what color to go with, maybe pink this time, next time, I would try the green one. It came in four colors, blue, green, pink, and yellow. It never occurred to me there was a difference in them, since I really didn't need deodorant. I wasn't much of a sweater. I just wanted to fit in, and I loved the name Tickle, since I was ticklish, and all of my friends used it. There was nothing like the feel of that huge wide ball under your arm. It was so wet, like a Great Dane licking your armpit. After each application, you had to walk around with your arms raised to let it dry, and you only had to just place it in your armpit since the ball was so big, and surprisingly enough, it didn't seem to go far. I was always back in the store, shopping for more, feeling as if everyone was watching what I was purchasing and thinking I must sweat a lot. Again, the name Tickle tickled me, and because of that, I had to have it.

When I moved to a bigger town, there was a drugstore. I loved going in this store. There were so many possibilities. When I got to the perfume aisle and saw that there were testers, I thought I'd won the lottery. It was hard to tell a smell though, after you have sprayed them all. Even though I never intended to buy any, I could not resist going in and getting a free spray now and then. I finally decided to purchase one for my mom for Mother's Day. It seemed like an elegant gift to give my mom for her special day. It is funny that thirty-two years later, she still has the same full bottle on her dresser. How sweet she decided to not use any, so she would have it forever.

I love shopping for nail polishes. The names are so fun. I wanted that job: having a single thought come to mind and no one overriding me, and all of a sudden, having a name for a polish. It felt so *Bewitched*, when Darin Stevens and Larry Tate were coming up with slogans. Believe me, I didn't need Samantha to come up with my own ideas. One that comes to mind: Slow dancing in Junior High.

MOVE YOUR HAIR PLEASE

We have all been there. Maybe at a movie, a play, even a baseball game. You get the perfect seat, so you think, and then the person in front of you sits down with big hair. You try to steer your line of vision around the side of them, but still, you cannot see. You lean to the other side, which is free for the moment, but the big hair just cannot stay stationary. You find an opening between the big hair and the object you are trying to view. The moment you can finally see, the big hair tilts, and your window is closed. You feel bad for the person seated behind you since you seem to not be able to make up your mind as to where to hold your head, but then you're sure they can see what is going on in front of you. If the big hair can be seen a couple of rows back, then it is time to rethink the hairdo. It is like having a top hat on, and a selfish fashion sense is making the rest of us miss what we have come to see. You spend a great deal of money for what you thought were great seats to something, not even thinking that your view could be blocked. There should be some sort of insurance you can purchase, in case you cannot see. Nothing like big hair blocking your view to ruin your big night out.

The person with the big hairdo has used the most amazing hairspray. The hairspray that would stop a fly in flight. If you were to light a match, the big hair would explode. You have such thoughts because it is so maddening. It is not going anywhere, but still, you want to take your hand, place it on the top of the hair tower, and smash it down, but then you run the risk of being escorted out. You sit and try to just listen to what is going on, occasionally checking the window. It is so distracting. You try not to focus on it, but you cannot help but stare at the back of it, dream of what you would like to do to it, all while missing the event you came to see. You are consumed by it. You run a few scenarios through your mind of a way that would fix this situation. Suddenly, the big hair is just that—as if a person is not attached to it and you want revenge. Then you tell yourself how you just want to see. Is that so bad?

When you go to a hair show, if you do not get there early, you could be faced to sit behind the sea of big hairs. Why do so many hair stylists have to have that big of hair? Must they use every product? I agree that products can be great and do just the thing your hair needs, but why so much lacquer? Shouldn't hair move? I think it should. If in a light wind storm, it should move a little. Making it tall on top is one thing, having a lot of lift, but does it also have to be so wide? Does it have to have that much volume? If your hair is wearing you, instead of the other way around, then you are in the wrong era, and you should take a seat in the back.

I once had a client who would come to see me for a shampoo and style when she was in town. She had the biggest hair, and I saw it on day seven, so you can imagine what it was like when it was freshly teased to high heavens. As the days wore on, the hair collapsed in a slow descend from all the added coats of hairspray.

She would tell me, in her New York accent, to "Tease it like there's no tama-rrow." I would too. I would just tease it, and her hair would stand on end, and I would just empty my can of hairspray onto it. She loved it, and it was exactly what she wanted. It made her look taller. She was five feet five, but with her teased hair, she was six feet! I wanted to send her out the back door, since I was embarrassed that I did that huge hairstyle. I guessed as long as she was happy with it, then I was too. She was the one who had to wear it, and she was parading out, sashaying to her ride in holy hairdo bliss.

Another client always says that back combing is like childbirth. In the middle of the strong heavy teasing and spraying, her face will hold a grimace. I tell her to do her breathing exercising, coach her along because she always says it is worth the pain. I let my arms rest from the workout, to make her feel better, let her know it was wearing me out, so her hair was not going anywhere for the next seven days. As I teased, I laughed and told her it was a double tease, so it was going to be even better.

I really don't have to sell my back-combing skills, though; they sell all on their own. After learning all of the roller sets in beauty school, I was really good at them. I got all of the little roller-set ladies in each week. I would roll one, put her under the dryer, wash and roll another, set her under the dryer, then comb one out, then the other, and then start the process over with two more roller-set ladies. This was how my days were being spent: doing roller sets. Every week was the same. I wanted more out of my career than doing roller sets. One night, I snuck my basket of rollers out and threw them in the garbage, as if throwing them away while it was dark outside would remain classified until I was ready to confess to my weekly roller-set clientele. I called all of my ladies to break the news that I would no longer be using the rollers, that they could still come in to see me, but I would use the progressive curling iron from then on. They all left me, but I was fine with it. I knew you didn't mess with the ladies of that era and their roller sets, but I was taking a stand. I didn't want to end up doing the same thing every day, every week. I wanted diversity.

I have worked with other stylists who have the same clients week after week, and they resent it. Especially Fridays, so the ladies can look good for the weekend. One stylist calls it "Cry Day." I then knew I had made the right decision about the roller disposal late that one dark night. Once you decide to throw your rollers in the garbage, you can never look back. The thing about the roller-set ladies is they knew exactly which way the roller was supposed to be placed. That decided the outcome. They only had one outcome in mind, and they wore it for a week, so if you weren't on the same page, it could be very stressful when you were combing out their hair. But if you could really back comb, then you have a roller-set client for life, if you want that.

NO TIME FOR LUNCH

We all have those days when our schedules are hectic. We don't have time for lunch, yet we are about ready to fall over from starvation. I always think that if I fall, I will try to fall away from my clients, so I will not stab them with my shears. I wouldn't want to wake up from a light-headed starvation pass-out moment and find that my client is in medical need. That is a bad way to lose business. I joke with my clients that they could hold my sandwich up, and I could take bites in between snips. This way, I could stay on schedule and wouldn't have to pick my sandwich up with wet, hairy hands. Also, I wanted to get one of those backpacks or hats that holds liquid so I could fill it up with a substantial protein drink that would help satiate my appetite until I could have a break. Usually, those devices were used at a tailgate party and were filled with beer, but I had taken a vow to never drink and cut.

The ol' drink and cut. I have heard stories from clients about their previous stylists who would indulge in alcohol before work, coming in smelling of booze. That has to be the worst feeling, to go for a haircut and find your stylist, the one holding the shears above you, intoxicated. Or just as bad, hungover, still smelling of the night before. You know they are not on their game, but they seem to have a lot more interesting ideas. There are clients who make me want to drink and cut, but I would never. I took an oath.

Some clients come in eating their lunch. I am fine with that, as long as I don't have to smell the aromas if I'm hungry. If I am applying the color, and they have to sit while they process, they will wait to eat their lunch then. For those who come in on their lunch break and are starving, I have snacks to get them by. I have a toaster in my studio, and sometimes my clients and I will have toast and tea together as they are processing their color. I am always making some toasted sandwich and then taking it into the break room, and my coworkers always ask where I got it. I tell them I made it in my studio. I have given clients crackers if they come in sick. One guy didn't want to cancel on me last minute, yet he was running to the bathroom to throw up. Have I put that much fear in them to not want to stand me up? Even though it tells me they respect me, I would understand upon the first look at their pale faces. Besides, clients who come in sick risk spreading it to me. One lady coughed in my face as I was leaning over her at the shampoo bowl. A week later, I caught her cold. Gee, I wonder how that happened.

I had another lady in recently who coughed up in my face as I shampooed her. By the time I responded to turning away from her, she got three coughs in, while her tongue curled out with each one. I leaned back as fast as I could and looked at myself right there in the mirror and mouthed, "What the..." A week later, I was sick. Do I really need to tell grown adults to cover their mouths when they cough?

A respectful male client called to tell me he would not make his afternoon appointment, that he was working outside and a branch hit his head. He was bleeding but thought he better cancel with me first, before he headed off to the emergency room.

Sometimes, even when you are hungry, you can lose your appetite on a gross scalp encounter. A flaky scalp can take away your lunch cravings. Although I do not work with many of these conditions, there have been a few occasions when I have had to skip a meal. One time, a preteen boy came in, and as he sat in my chair, I noticed how greasy his hair was. I told him to follow me, so we could shampoo his hair. He just sat there and started to cry. I asked him if he was crying because I was going to shampoo his hair. He said that he was. I told him it would be OK; I would be very careful. He didn't want to do it and just sat there, so I just sprayed him down with the water bottle, making a huge mistake since his hair was so dirty. I should have refused his service since it appeared he hadn't washed his hair in weeks, making my hands smell of dirty head. I had to sit in the break room during my lunch break with a layer of dish soap all over my hands to try to get that smell out of them. Nothing makes you lose your desire to eat more than that smell as you bring your hand up to your mouth with a bite. The next time the kid was on my schedule, I called his mom to tell her he needed to let me shampoo his hair first or I would not cut his hair. Losing him was the best thing for my stomach.

BETTER HIDE THE SHEARS

There was one time when I did fear for my life. I had only had my hair license for about three months and started working in a little salon in a strip mall. I was there, doing a little boy's haircut, when this man walked in and wanted a haircut. I was the only stylist working, so I told him I could cut his hair in fifteen minutes. As I started thinking about it, knowing I would be alone with him all tucked into the back of the salon, I started to get nervous.

I talked to the mom of the little boy about it, and she said she would call the salon to check on me in twenty minutes. As they left, the pit in my stomach started to grow, and the man followed me back to my station. All I could think about was how we were there alone. He seemed creepy, but maybe it was the actual situation making me feel that way. His hair was short, military style, and in that era, you only had that style of cut if you were or had been in the service. He was rambling on and could not decide what he wanted. There was not much I could do since it was already short.

Finally, the phone rang, and I went to answer it. I quickly grabbed my shears for fear he would stab me with them. I just knew it would happen, since my mom took such precaution in preparing me for such events. How many times would I be tested and thrown a stranger to stir up some fear in me? When I answered the phone, it was the mom, and she was checking up on me. I said I was OK and then hung up. Well, so far I was OK, but what then? Was that all the checking up on I got? I should have told her to call me in another twenty minutes. I was feeling so alone, as if no one in the world knew what was going on in this little tucked away mini-mall hair shop. I was there all alone with some psychopathic killer. I hid all of my sharp objects before I led him back to my station, just in case he was unstable and was being good at hiding it in front of my last clients.

When I finally finished, I walked him out to the front to collect his money. He complained about the price, but paid me. No tip, although I stayed late, risking my life for his hair. He looked in the mirror above the desk and said something about having more taken off. I told him there was nothing more to cut. You know, once the cape is off and you are out of the chair, that window is closed, you missed your chance to have more taken off. That is, your time is up if you are a psycho, and I am ready to get you out the salon before you attack me. I will take more off a good client. If a good client goes home, plays with it a week and calls for more taken off, I will gladly take more off, no extra charge.

As he walked toward the door, my heart was pounding. I just wanted him to leave, and I wanted to feel safe. He opened the door, then stood there looking at me. The thing going through my mind was hopefully he liked my haircut and would spare me. Yes, my cutting capabilities would save my life. He wanted my business card. Did I even tell him my name? Could I pass off someone else's business card as my own? I just grabbed one and handed it to him. As he finally left, I leaped and locked the door. He watched me do it and tried to open the door again. I told him he had to leave, that I had somewhere to be...inside, without him. I walked to the back of the salon to clean up and would not go home for a good hour, hoping he was gone. I had a feeling that told me to wait, so I listened.

I decided to never put myself in that position again. Was the money really worth the stress? Was I really in trouble with that guy? I wasn't certain. I just knew that coming from a small town, we learned to never trust a stranger. I had to listen to my inner whisper, and it was telling me to be on my toes. The feeling was different if the person was friendly. The guy never smiled, making him seem unkind, unstable somehow. I am better these days with my intuition and have learned to trust it.

If I am going to be locked in and the last person leaving before me asks me if I want to be locked in, I will ask myself if I want to be locked in with the client presently in my chair. I had a frisky male client in one night, and the person leaving before me asked me if I wanted her to lock the door.

I asked out loud, "Hmmm, let me see. Is that a trick question? Do I want to be locked in with so and so?" We all just laughed.

The Falling Shears

Our shears are expensive. We hate to drop them and ruin them, maybe breaking off the tip, or getting them out of alignment. One time, a coworker, while dropping her shears, put out her leg to break their fall, and as they fell down, they sliced her leg. That was a lesson for all of us.

Still, we hate to have them fall to the hard floor, so we try to protect them. My shears were falling once, so I went to grab them. As I put my hands out to catch them, with my eyes closed, I noticed that they didn't hit the floor and opened my eyes to see where they landed. They were stuck in my wrist, jammed in there by a prominent vein. I pulled them out and waited for the blood to gush, but it never did. I felt woozy, and my client told me to sit down. It was a lucky day for me indeed. The shear went in, the dull side against the vein, so I was going to live. I did have to go to the doctor to have a tetanus shot. I have the scar that reminds me to let the shears fall if they are going to fall, or to be more careful, putting them in a safer place when they are not in use. Otherwise, there could be a fatal accident. My problem was that I was always in a hurry and had to rush out to get my kids from day care by a certain time, or the day-care facility would charge a dollar a minute. That was hard when your last client of the day was late. You couldn't rush beauty, but there were many times when I had to race out to get the kids and come back to the salon to clean up. A couple of times, I swept the pile of hair under my mat, and that was against my OCD tendencies.

I had a shears holster. When I first got it, I wore it all the time. I felt like Quick Draw McGraw. When I was done with my shears, I would blow on them, as if they were a smoking gun, carefully twirl them around my thumb, and holster them as fast as I could. My clients laughed. The novelty wore off, and I didn't wear it for years. It made me feel so ready. Ready to cut at any given notice. It was good to always be ready for a hair duel. Plus, the holster was nice, since I always had my tools on my person, in case someone decided to make off with them. I have had so many things taken from my station. I would come to work, open my color cabinet, and there would be tubes of color gone. I have a system for storing my hair color. I start with the darkest color (one) and go up the lightest color (ten) and then have my high-lift colors after that. One day, I came to work, and the numbers were out of order. When I pushed the six series color up, I could see what color was missing. Of course, I wrote a note on the board in the break room, which was there for anyone feeling passive aggressive but never solved anything. The next day, another stylist asked me to show her how I stored my color, and as I was showing her, the missing color was back. Someone went to the supply house and replaced it, probably since I made a big deal out of it. It was a big deal. If you are an independent contractor, you need to run your business. It isn't fair that I go to the supply house every week to make sure I am stocked, and then someone can just come in and help themselves when they want. I would open my drawer and find a full bottle of peroxide gone, and I would get the same things said to me, "Are you sure?" "Yes! I am sure!" I knew I needed to work in a place where I could lock it up at night, so no one could help themselves. The day someone stole my pink baby stapler and all the extra staples with it—that one sent me over the edge. To me, it meant that someone was very familiar with my drawers and knew it was there. If anyone ever asked me to borrow something, I would always say yes: a birthday candle, gum, whatever, but don't steal my baby stapler. I knew it would never be returned since the box of extra staples was also missing.

I told some of my coworkers, and they said, "Are you sure? Who would steal a stapler?"

"Yes, I am sure," and that was when I knew I had to find a new salon.

When I went to see my friend who had just started at Sola Salon Studios, I walked in just to see her studio and drop off a gift. What I didn't expect was to feel so taken in and at home. A feeling came over me, and I just knew I had to work there. I said goodbye to my friend and had every intention to leave, but as I was walking around looking at all of the studios, I was falling deeper in love. One of the stylists came out of her studio to ask me if I needed help. I told her I was just visiting a friend who had just started working there and that I was looking around. She invited me to look at her studio and was telling me how she loved working there. I went back to my friend, and at first, she was shocked I was still there. She thought I had left forty minutes prior. I told her I was talking with stylists and looking at studios, and that I had to work there as well. She texted the manager with my name and contact info, and three days later, I was offered a studio. I was in shock since I heard it was hard to get into Sola. There was a waiting list with seven stylists ahead of me, but they wanted other Sola stylists to refer people they knew, so I was able to take the next available studio. What an exciting moment it was! But the other side was having to give your month's notice and then live in the salon you were leaving for that month.

The move has been the best thing for me. It is my home away from home, and I have made it so comfortable and inviting. When you lease a studio from Sola, you get to name your studio, choose the paint color, and decorate as you like. I chose the name H202. I asked my clients if they knew what it meant, and some of them did. It is peroxide, and since I use peroxide for hair color, I thought it was fitting. I joke with my clients that I was thinking about naming it Debbie's Beauty Barn and that I could have a bale of hay instead of a couch. When I didn't laugh right away, I think they believed me.

I am contained in my studio with a coffeepot, tea, and water, and I have a refrigerator with snacks and a toaster if we want to toast something. I have a TV as well, and I say how I could spend the night there when the weather was bad. I did take a nap one day when I had a two-and-a-half-hour cancellation. I pulled my curtains, turned the lights out, asked Alexa to play James Taylor music, and curled up on my couch with the blanket. It is a good feeling to know I can do this, and I wonder if everyone is wondering if I am in there, maybe napping. The nice thing about it is that I don't have to hide anything anymore, since I know that when I come to work, everything will still be where I left it.

WEIRDO IN THE CHAIR

I have had more than my share of questionable clients who give me the creeps. I think I have good instincts, but I need to be more faithful in listening to them. When you are first starting out, you have to take every client you can get—anyone who walks in the door—so you can build your clientele. Even if the weirdo may not like his hair or even care what it looks like. Maybe a neighbor or family member will notice, and the word will spread about you and your cutting talents.

I had a client who started out normal, but things took a turn when I became single. He would show up for a haircut appointment with "treats" for me, such as a couple scoops of ice cream with two spoons. Did he actually think I was going to take my break after cutting his hair to share the ice cream with him? How sweet, the two of us sitting outside, enjoying the sun and sharing cookies and cream. It wasn't even my flavor. What a creep! He could have at least asked me what I liked. I would have told him a scoop of espresso and cream and mint chocolate chip, but then he would know something too personal about me.

He would also bring things like a boiled egg, peeled, in a baggy. What makes someone think, "Oh, I have a haircut today. I will bring her a boiled egg. First, I shall peel it." Of course, it went right into the garbage, but not in front of him because my good manners tend to take over at times. I excused myself when he first came in and took it to the back, saying I wanted to put it in the refrigerator, but threw it in the trash. Why couldn't I just say that was a strange thing? Why did he bring it? I wanted to know. Maybe I looked as if I needed more protein.

He used to tell me how he dreamed of my magic fingers while I was washing his hair. Great way to get the massage cut short. I barely did a full lather, since I was afraid he would say more. Or worse…moan. That is a weird thing that can happen while you are shampooing, to have someone moan. I have had a client purr as a joke, but to actually start moaning and mean it. I know this because their eyes are closed and they are continuing to do it, even though I am onto them. I heard it and was trying to decide if I should stop short, maybe hit the client with some cooler water during the final rinse to wake them up. Are they in la-la land? Are they pretending they are somewhere else? It is OK to let me know how much they like the shampoo, and by that, I mean they can let me know through being quiet and staying in a restful state. There is no need to moan as if it were a reenactment of the deli scene from *When Harry Met Sally.* That takes it to another level I do not want to visit. I do not want what you are having.

I couldn't even turn him to face the mirror, since he would make comments that left me uncomfortable. I never wanted to give it away that he got to me. I played it cool, pretended not to care. I really didn't care what he thought; I just didn't want to deal with his come-ons anymore. He sent his mother in to get her hair done with me, and she went on and on about her son. I was polite, said nothing, and let her glorify him. I started to wonder if her son told her we were dating, since she was acting as if we were family. I was starting to worry she would invite me for the holidays.

He would come in and tell me about his new jeep, even wanted to show me and take me for a ride. I knew if I were to get in his jeep, he would never bring me back. I looked at it from the door of the salon to be polite, waved goodbye, thought about how I would have to deal with this again in another four weeks, if he didn't drop by earlier with some treat for me. I knew I had to put an end to it, so I started charging PITA, cut the shampoo, and was done in half the time.

One time, when I was pregnant and on my own, he told me he wanted to be my labor coach. There was no way I was going to let him consider this for a minute. I would not want to see him in the delivery room, down there, watching my baby being born, or even holding my hand, telling me to breathe while feeding me ice chips. He was not going to be any focal point. Who was this guy, and why did he think he had a front-row seat to my life? I was certainly not leading him on in any way.

He did bring me a chocolate éclair while I was pregnant. My first response was to throw it away, but as the sweet smell rose to my nose, I had enough sense to at least save it and reconsider eating it after he was gone. I liked to think my cravings got the best of me. I told him I hid it on top of the refrigerator in the break room. After he left, I went back to get it, and it was gone! There were only a few stylists working that morning. No one was back there when I "hid" it on top of the fridge, behind the stack of paper towels. Now, more than ever, I wanted it. I looked all around for it, even checking the garbage for the doily it was on, but it was not there. I checked in all of the cupboards, no éclair. I asked all of the other stylists, while checking for traces of chocolate on the corners of their mouths, but no one had seen it. That was when my craving really hit and I started to panic. The first time the weirdo brought me something I liked, I hid it and now it was gone.

Now I knew how my mother felt when she said it didn't just grow legs and walk off! Another stylist got up on the counter to check on top of the refrigerator for me. She came in as I was beginning to climb on the chair. I guess a pregnant woman shouldn't climb up on a chair, but I thought the éclair was calling for me from up there. We never found it, and it was the salon mystery for years. It didn't make me like him more. In fact, I was upset with him for tempting me with sweets, and to this day, I have never had an éclair.

The same client, Mr. Boiled Egg, I will call him, worked in a grocery store as a checker. I would avoid him, but he would always find me and pull my cart to his line and make comments on the contents I was buying. Very undesirable when it was feminine hygiene products. He told me about how they used to use cotton and gauze in World War I and so on, since they didn't have tampons or pads. It was so uncomfortable and wrong. I was standing there, shaking my head while asking him to stop talking about it. Another time, I was in another checker's line and his phone rang. The checker then told me the phone was for me. This was the phone only the checkers used, stationed at their registers. It was him, telling me I should have gone through his line. He even blocked me in one time at the gas station, calling my name and waving. It was very creepy. Was he following me, or did he just happen to be in the same vicinity as me? How lucky was I?

He sent me a Christmas card that alarmed me. It said "I look forward to the hour a month that you hold sharp implements near my neck." What really did this mean? It made me feel uneasy, I will tell you that. I told several of my guy friends about it; I also shared where he worked. They went to pay this grocery store checker a visit, went through his line, and let him know they knew me, giving him the look. This made me feel better that others knew what I was going through with him and that they were looking out for me.

Just when I thought he was gone, he came back. Wouldn't you know, my prices went up again. When he asked how much he owed, I told him, and he commented that I had really raised my prices.

I said, "Yes, I have two kids to feed."

He said, "I can't help that you pop them out left and right." OK, that was it. There was no way this man was ever sitting in my chair again. I told him how rude he was and asked him to leave. The last time I saw him at the grocery store and he took me into his line, I had my daughter with me. She was the one he wanted to "coach" during birth.

I said, "Oh, this is my daughter. I popped her out left, or was it right?" I was thankful that was the last time I ever saw him. I talked to his manager that night, telling of how he said gross things as he rang up items, giving him examples. He was either fired or relocated. Hopefully he was not tormenting some other young, starving hair stylist, trying to feed her boiled eggs and share ice cream. An éclair would be all right, but only during pregnancy.

DERRIERE AWARENESS

One thing you must have when you work in a salon, is derriere awareness. It is when you are bending over sweeping or picking up something from the floor—any bending, really—and you know to point your derriere *away* from the client, toward a wall, perhaps, away from his or her line of vision. This helps to avoid the underwear moment. You know the one. You have seen it all exposed above the waistband of the pants. This is a perimeter that it should not cross, for the waistband is a sacred barrier.

I worked with a girl whose station was a few feet away from mine. She would sweep, and when it came time to use the dustpan, she would bend by my client's arm and expose her underwear. This was a straight leg bend, so it was right in my client's face, not near the floor where it should have taken place. At first, I dismissed it, thinking she didn't realize what she was doing, but as time went on, it happened upon every sweeping session. I learned to turn my clients away at that crucial moment. Once, I had a young man in. I wanted to see how he would respond. He was in the middle of telling me a story...I saw the broom in use, and as he turned to look, he saw that her derriere was right by his arm, inches away, by the armrest of the chair. A bright pink thong was sticking up out of her black slacks. He was speechless. I then discreetly give him the look that told him I knew what was going on. Other times, I told my clients to wait for it, and then I'd turn them in the direction of the action and let them witness it, and then I would whisper in the client's ear, "She doesn't have derriere awareness."

Another time, she was all bent over at the front desk, showing a little butt crack. She was talking about how she had been on vacation.

My client was seated behind her behind in the reception area, her backside near his face, and when the time was right, he told her how he was "happy to see her back." She didn't get it. It was priceless. How do you not feel all exposed back there? You know when you are flashing some butt crack. You can feel the breeze. Who are you kidding? Do you really want us to see it? We are going to look. It's like the eclipse, you shouldn't look at it, but you just cannot help yourself.

Whenever I see it, I say, "Look at the BC" (butt crack).

I live on a main street, so I have to be aware of my derriere at all times. When I go out to get the morning paper, I don't just bend over, rear to the road. I bend at the knee, point my derriere toward the garage, and have some consideration for the passersby. Sometimes, I am in the middle of pulling a tough weed and notice a car headed my way. I struggle with the weed, maybe call it a name, and then as the car gets closer, I have to point my derriere the other way and let up on it. Once they have passed, I am back at the weed, and it's going to get it. I always use the polite approach. This technique works well in the salon and is much more classy.

How about at the grocery store? You are minding your own business, turn your cart on a particular aisle, and then you are face-to-face with it. Right in front of you, blocking the entire aisle, is a derriere bending over, as if saying, "Here I am...look at me."

The only thing it is missing is a big target. You cannot get around it, and it is not letting you by until it has what it has bent over to get. For some reason, you cannot get by it. It has to take up the whole passing space with the cart, and then the bending over motion. It is rude on many levels, and for some reason, this is not a quick ritual. They do it, taking their time, as if it were a yoga pose they had to hold.

That is when I say to myself, "They don't have derriere awareness."

The last big hair show I went to, I should have shared this knowledge with some of the stylists on the stage. First of all, the look is not good when the shirt looks too small and the pants are a low-rise, when you are on stage, demonstrating a haircutting technique, bending over, derriere to the audience, and you are showing your whale tail. If you choose to wear a thong, you shouldn't show it off to the world if you are not in shape and your roll is hanging over the top of your waistline. Again, how can you not feel all this hanging out? You know you will have your hands up in the haircutting position and will be on stage. Some mornings, as I am getting ready for work and trying to put an outfit together, I do the test and lift my arms to see how high the shirt rises up and how low the pants are, so I will not have that awkward moment when I am trying to reach a part of the hair that needs my arms in that position. I always want to be prepared. Do these people not think out their stage outfits, or do they just not care? It is a mystery. Maybe some people like it. I am not a fan. It is hard for me to focus on haircutting when all of that is going on.

Someone will ask me what I learned from the show, and I will answer, "I learned how to not dress when you have my profession and to be aware of your derriere at all times.

I had a dad and son in who were getting haircuts. The little boy was sitting in a chair off to the side. I had my back to him at one point. I was working with the clipper, so I was slightly bent, checking out the dad's hairline.

I heard the little boy say, "Nice view there, with your butt in my face." I quickly turned to face him and he had scooted the chair up, very close to me, so as I bent over to check my work, my derriere was sort of in the vicinity of his face, and he was letting me know. I could not stop laughing. I kept telling him I was sorry and that I didn't know he moved his chair so close.

The dad was so embarrassed, he kept telling his son to move back, and then the little boy said again, "Well, it was just in my face." I was mortified. The next time I saw them, the little boy said, "I am not going to mention anything about last time when your butt was in my face." I guessed his dad talked to him, but he couldn't help himself. He had to say something. It was good that he would learn an important lesson so young, so he could carry it with him throughout his years and have manners.

Sometimes, the comb would fall when I was cutting the client's hair. If it is in the back, it will fall to the floor, no problem, so you get a new one. If it is in the front and lands in the lap, it could seemingly drop in slow motion, coming to rest in the client's lap. One time, it was falling, and I watched as it fell down the front of the client. I tried to grab, but decided to let it go, since I was afraid I would grab something I should not grab.

I just watched it as it grazed his lap, and then watched it land on the floor, and I said, "I thought it best not to grab." We started laughing. One time, I had a new lady in my chair, and as the comb started to fall, I grabbed it and grabbed her breast! I caught the comb on her breast, and when it registered to me that my hand was on the comb, on her breast, I quickly let go and the comb fell to the floor. I had a moment of silence, since I wasn't sure how to handle it. Well, I did handle it, her breast, and then my face was turning red. I very quickly said I was sorry, that I was trying to grab the comb.

When she left, I walked over to the stylist across the hall and said, "I grabbed a breast!" We had a little chuckle, and I was reminded of how I should always let the comb fall. You don't want the client thinking you are inappropriate, or coming onto them, and I have a drawer full of combs. What is the five-second rule on that? I wait five seconds, and if I feel I cannot grab it, I let it fall to the floor and then get a new one. If it falls and remains in the client's lap, I wait a few seconds, hoping the client will retrieve it and hand it back. Again, I don't want to seem forward to grab at anything I should not be grabbing and make them think I am getting frisky with them.

The lady came back for a second appointment, and all I could think about was not to drop the comb and grab her breast. I did drop the comb, but I jumped back, hands in the air, sort of letting her know I would not make the same mistake twice. It sounds as though I drop the comb a lot, but I think I drop it a normal amount. I will have to take a poll and get back to you.

I had a lady in who was processing her hair color. I was on my couch, having a little snack. She told me a story about falling down outside while she was pressure washing, and told me to close my curtains and my door. I wanted to finish my lunch, but she was insisting on closing up the shop. As I was closing the curtains and turned back around, I saw she had her pants pulled down and her bottom was exposed.

She said, "Do you see that?" I wasn't sure what I was supposed to be seeing.

There was a mole and a wart on her left butt cheek, so I said, "What am I supposed to be seeing?" She pointed to the bruise on the other cheek, which was black and blue. I said, "That looks terrible, but you may want to get the other things checked."

Six months later, she was in my chair and said, "I had a wart." I asked her where it was. She said it was on her left backside.

I said, "I told you that you should get that checked." Now, whenever I walk past a studio that has the curtains drawn, I assume they are viewing a bottom.

RULES TO ABIDE BY

We do not, as hair stylists, have many rules. We are very easy to get along with. I don't think I have a mean bone in my body. Sure, I try to sound all tough, but really, deep down, I am just a softie. One rule that can really set me off, besides grabbing my bottom, or any groping really, is when a client wipes the color on the cape he or she is wearing. You want to wear your glasses while your color is processing. You take them off and wipe them off on the cape. It is a bad choice. First of all, you have now gotten color on the cape, so it may get on you. Secondly, it may now get on the chair, and another client may sit in it, or lean against it. We, as stylists, are liable. Plus, our capes are expensive, and we want to keep them nice for you. If you have a color-wiping need, just say so, and I will give you a towel. I have purchased eyeglass condoms, which fit over the temple tips of the glasses, protecting them from color. I think you should always use protection when coloring.

One time, a client went to town wiping off her glasses on the cape, and as she stood, it was all over the front of the cape. I got a bit snippy with her about it, pointing out the "color scene" and told her how it ruined the cape. It would stain it, and then I would only bring it out on that client's visit, making her wear the ugly stained cape to see how she liked it. If a client was done processing, and we were getting ready to shampoo, the minute he or she took his or her glasses off, I was on it. Otherwise, the client was so quick to start using the cape to remove the color from the temples of the glasses. I took the glasses and told the client I would clean them. By now, I have my clients pretty well trained, and they either take their glasses to my sink to wash them or use a Kleenex, but they know I will wash the color off for them.

Also, if you forgo your glasses and just want to rest your eyes, make sure you don't lean if you are under the dryer. You may fall asleep and use the dryer hood to hold up your head. This is not a good idea if you are getting a foil weave. You may cause the foils to slip, and the color will bleed onto your scalp, leaving a bleached line. Please take note, and accept the coffee I have offered you.

Please Be Courteous and Turn off Your Cell Phone

Doing hair when clients are on the phone is hard. First of all, they tilt their heads, holding one shoulder up higher, so they are not sitting straight. Getting around the ear is hard. There is no way you are going to bend it because they are already bending the ear of the listener on the other end of the line. A client will bring his or her phone in, leaving it in a bag, and the minute it rings, jump up to get it. I could be in the middle of an important cut, the one that decides the outcome, but he or she will leap to the phone, without any regard as to what I am doing. When the client is seated again, I have to comb and find that spot again, and get it just right. It is so rude. I know it can be an important call, and I understand, but not when he or she is just talking on and on about nothing. If you are expecting an important call, give me a heads up; keep your phone within reach, so you don't have to bolt from the chair the minute you hear your ring tone. You cannot help but listen to the conversation the client is having; you are right there as a captive audience, in his or her bubble.

Sometimes, clients on the phone will say, "Oh nothing. Just getting a haircut." If this is really nothing, then don't complain when it is uneven or it takes longer. Every time the client leans forward to reach for a phone, the cape goes with him or her, so when the client sits back, I have to pull the cape out again and tuck it on the outside of the chair. Sometimes, I try to grab it as he or she is leaning, so I can just put it back where I want it and not have to fish it out as the client is pressed up against it. I want to install a hook on the back of the chair so I can loop the cape on it, so he or she cannot lean forward. If the client is repeatedly leaning, and I am having to continually stop to fix the cape, I will ask him or her to please keep the phone in his or her lap. I recently saw a cape that had a clear, square window in the front so the client could have his or her phone under the cape and still see it. I think it would be a great idea for clients who like to "knit" as well, so I can always see what was going on.

Some clients like to come in to the salon to relax, to get away from things such as the phone. I don't stand there, cutting your hair while talking on my phone. It wouldn't be a good idea, since you have to raise your shoulder to keep the phone in place, and your head is at a slant. How are you going to cut a straight line when your head isn't aligned? I put my phone away. Maybe if I have to take a call, I will tell the client that I have an important call to take before we get started, and if it rings, I make it quick.

You would never hear from me, "Oh nothing. Just doing a haircut." The shears are down. I am not trying to multitask. At times, a client will leave their phone behind while he or she is being shampooed, and then the rest of us have to listen to it ringing.

One of my clients came in on the phone. I greeted him, and he followed me to my station, remaining on the phone. After draping him, I motioned for him to follow me, and we walked to the shampoo bowl. While I was waiting for him to hang up, I guided his head to the lean-back position, and it was time to turn the water on. I used to wait, but now, if his phone gets wet, his phone gets wet. He is on my time. This usually gets him to say goodbye to the other party.

I was coloring a guy's hair once, and he was talking on the phone while under the dryer, during the processing stage of the color. One of the sides of his hair did not take the color like the other side. I thought it was strange since I applied it evenly to both sides. It then dawned on me that he must have been on his phone. I looked at his phone and there was the color evidence.

The next time his color was processing, I said, "Hand it over," and made him give his phone to me. I told him it was a no-phone color zone and that he needed to properly process. One time, he tried to sneak it, but I was aware of the situation. Sometimes, when he is not looking, and it is sitting on my counter, I will hide it. It is not a bad thing that I want his color to turn out on both sides.

When it is time to blow-dry, and if the client is still on his or her phone, I am no longer waiting for him or her to get off before I turn the dryer on. I used to wait until clients were done, but I have a schedule to keep as well, and I do not allow more time for the use of a phone. If they are on a call, I will clean up and let them talk, but when I am done cleaning and sweeping around them, I am ready to dry their hair, so it is time to end the call.

I had a client in who would use his cell phone during the entire appointment. I would tap him on the shoulder and point for him to switch ears so I could work on the other side, but it's too hard to really judge the evenness of the hair. He would always go into the bathroom and inspect the cut for what seemed like ten minutes. During this time, I didn't know what to do. I would clean and get ready for my next client, who would be out in the waiting room, and I would find myself pacing, waiting to see if he approved of my work. One day, in particular, he had been on his phone the whole haircut time, making me run late, so I went and got my next client, not awaiting the ten-minute inspection outcome. He finally came out of the bathroom and pointed out that one side wasn't quite even with the other side.

I told him, "That was your phone ear." He just looked at me, as if I was being unfair that his time was up and I had glossed over him. I was not going to invest any more time on him since he could not have phone respect. It was my time too, and if you want me to do a good job, please be courteous and turn off your phone!

How about when you are done with your clients and they now want to show you all of their vacation pictures or a long video? Some days are just busier than others, and I don't always have time to look at every picture. I am glad they want to share with me, but it is usually the clients who were late who want to do this. I have had moments of wondering to myself what they would think if I took their phones and threw them down the hall. These thoughts make me laugh, and I call them coping mechanisms. It is just the thinking of doing it that calms my nerves. Sort of like when you are at the grocery store and another patron is just standing there with his or her cart in the middle of the aisle, and even though the individual sees you trying to get by, he or she ignore you and continues to look at a shopping list. Well, I wish I could ram the person's cart with mine, not that I would, but the mere thought of it makes me feel better. It makes me think we need more rules. Plus, the phone is taking over our lives, and we should learn to unplug and enjoy the luxury of getting our hair done without jumping up to retrieve it whenever it rings.

THE SLEEPER

We all know how relaxing it can be when you are having your hair done. First of all, you are sitting still, with no agenda at that moment. How often in the day do you get to just sit? It makes you tired. You are sitting, you had a nice scalp massage, and you're getting your hair combed through, starting to get sleepy. I can usually detect this. I used to take offense to it, thinking maybe I was boring, causing them to doze. Now, I take it as a compliment. I know the sleeper must trust me, or he or she would be awake and aware.

I have a client who always dozes off. I look for the long blinks, then the eyes close and he starts to drop his head forward. Usually a loud noise would cause him to stir, sit up for a moment, and then fall asleep again! I usually tell my coworkers to be quiet, since my client is trying to nap. Now that I am in a studio by myself, it is quiet and ideal for his haircutting sleep session.

When the sleepy client is sleeping and leaning, I have to really bend to be able to cut his hair. I do have to move his head to the proper position so I can see to cut his hair. I would hate to van Gogh him, since he hasn't given me any reason not to let him leave with both ears intact. He says the clippers make him sleepy, but I think he has dozed off well before the clippers were in use. I tell him he should get some clippers to use as a white noise machine at night if he is having a hard time sleeping, but for some reason, I don't think it is a problem for him, unless he is dozing in my chair because he cannot sleep at night and needs to go to the sleep clinic for a night to figure this out. When I am getting close to finishing, I will tap him on the shoulder to let him know I need him to wake up and sit upright, as if he were flying and it was time to return to the landing position. Once I tried to cut his sideburns while his head was down, and when he did sit up, they were at a slant. I learned that I should never cut the sideburns when the head is down. Always wake your client before you do the final edging. A light spritz from the water bottle does the job. One time, he was really leaning, and I was having a hard time getting him to stay upright, so I kept spraying my water bottle in the air over him, hoping the cool water mist would rouse him. He opened his eyes, and I acted as if I was just spraying a section, and not just full throttling it above his head. He told me that when he went on vacation, he had to have a hair affair since he was gone for so long, and it stressed him out, having a stranger cut his hair. He said he couldn't sleep at all, so it was a compliment to me.

One day, when he was really sleeping, his head was so bent over, it gave me the giggles. It was April Fool's Day, and I thought about going back and having my lunch while he rested. I wondered if he would know I was gone. The thought of him waking and wondering where I had gone was making me laugh. Every once in a while, he would wake; I thought maybe he felt me shaking while I was laughing, and I had to act natural, as if I wasn't even on to him that he was asleep. Sometimes I worry as he leaves and think, *Is he safe to drive?* Would he wake up before he was on the road? A client once told me there should be a room to go relax in after you had your hair done, and maybe get some orange juice and a cookie to get your energy back up before you get behind the wheel.

Dream a Little Dream

I know I am not alone when I say I have dreams about my clients. It is very embarrassing when it is a sexual dream. Do you tell them or not? Not! It stays with you for a while. You tell some of your coworkers, even tell them the client will be in at 2:15 p.m., to make sure they get a good look at the one who starred in your dream.

I had a client in my dream who had a nice head of hair. I dreamed he had a single gray hair in the middle of his forehead. I mentioned this obviously misplaced single hair to him, and he told me to pull it (If only this wasn't a dream; I could have told him about my one buck pluck). I wanted to cut it, but he insisted I pull it, so I gave it a yank, but it still didn't come out. His head moved along with the yanking of the hair followed by an "Ouch!" Once again, he asked me to pull it. I wrapped the hair around my finger and pulled it again, but still, it would not budge. I was determined to pull this hair that didn't belong, so I wrapped a wet towel around the hair and really gave it a tug, but his head again moved along with the hair, and the hair remained. I was laughing in the dream, although I knew I should not laugh, and then I woke up laughing and had a little tickle about it all day.

Usually, I have stress dreams where my client is at the salon, waiting for me, but I cannot get there. I try to call, but I keep misdialing. Once, I was swimming in the fast lane on the freeway and just could not crawl fast enough to get to work. If only I had a wall to push off from. When I have such a vivid dream like that, I wake up so exhausted, since I was so busy swimming down I-5. Sometimes, I will dream I have a few clients in at once, and I need to finish because I have more coming in. I am not sure what all of this means, but I like to think it is because I always try to go above and beyond for my clients. I like to give them my undivided attention, providing them a good service, and that starts with being on time.

I often have dreams that when the clients are having their hair shampooed, they are in a bed. Maybe it is because they are somewhat lying down and relaxed. I did dream that while my client was relaxed in bed, I was coloring his gray chest hairs. It is weird when you wake up and take a moment to think about it and then realize that person is on your schedule that day. You are a little embarrassed to face the client, even though he or she is clueless. I have no idea why I dream some of the things I do, but we are not accountable for our dreams, and it does happen. Sweet dreams!

WAKING UP ON THE WRONG
SIDE OF THE HEAD

I am usually aware of where clients part their hair. Only about 15 percent part it on the right and comb it to the left, since most people are right handed, or if they have a cowlick and are forced to wear it to the left. Fighting the cowlick is not best, but make peace with the way it wants to lay. This statistic makes it easy. Since I do cut the hair neutrally, it can go either way, but I want to make sure to send them out with their hair going the way they usually wear it.

I have a client who I have been cutting for eighteen years. For fourteen of the years, after the haircut, I have been combing it to the right and sending him on his way. He reschedules, does not say one word, even gives me a hug. Four years ago, while he was sitting in my chair, for some reason, I noticed his hair was combed to the left. I guessed the chair was in the lowest position, and I could really get a good look down upon his head. I questioned this, asking if he had changed his part.

He said, "No, Dear. You are the one who parts it the other way. I wear it out and then the next day, comb it the other way." He said it looked good both ways because I cut it so he can wear it either way, but I was amazed that I missed this. Me. Nothing goes unnoticed with me. I am usually on top of these matters. He reassured me it was a sign of a good haircut, since it was so versatile.

I did cut a guy's hair once who was watching me style his hair. I got all the way to the end, just about ready to take the cape off, and he said his hair normally went on the other side. He had been watching me the entire time, without a word about his part. It is harder to get it to go the other way once you have dried it, using a nice strong gel to keep it in place. So I had to take him to the shampoo bowl again, wet it down and style it the other way. If your hair is on the wrong side, just say the word and I would be happy to change it before it's time to take the cape off.

One guy told me he left his stylist because she couldn't remember where his part was. Hearing this made me want to pay special attention. I took a mental picture at the shampoo bowl because I didn't want to "part" ways with a client because I left them parted on the wrong side of the head.

MORE TEARS BEHIND
THE CHAIR

A client once told me a sad story about his dog passing away. He stopped in the beginning of his story and told me he decided not to tell me since I might cry. I joked about how I had a box of Kleenex and that I would be fine. I thought I could handle it, but it turned out that I could not control myself. He sat there, telling me the story of the last day he'd had with his dog, how he had gone to the vet, and they had suggested the dog be euthanized, but he had decided to wait and had taken the dog to his favorite spot down by the river, where he'd carried him to their spot, and then my lip quivered as I fought back tears. At the end of the story, he told me he was going to take him to the vet to be put to sleep, but the dog died in his arms as they got back in the pickup. I lost it and had to excuse myself and go into the bathroom to have a moment. I told a coworker why I was crying, and she said she would cry too, making me cry more. I had to get myself together and had my coworker go tell my client I needed a minute and would be right back to finish his haircut.

Another client was telling me about the passing of her cat. It was such a touching story; it felt as if I were right there with her and the cat until the end. I started to tear up and told her that I couldn't see to cut her hair with the pool of tears in my eyes.

At least I was the one crying in the chair...

One of my longest clients was coming in before she was moving out of state. Toward the end of the cut, I started feeling sad that she was moving away, that it was possibly the last time she would be in my chair. I had to leave her a few times to wipe my tears. While she was gone, I thought of her around her five-week appointment mark and wondered how she was doing and if she was surviving her new hair stylist. Then, after eight weeks passed, I got a call from her, and she told me she was moving back, after only one hair affair. Technically, it was not a hair affair, since I knew it was going to happen. I believe she moved back because she could not find anyone to do her hair like I did. And now, I shall excuse myself, for my head is getting too big, and it is getting hard to see the keyboard. She mentioned she was thinking about moving again. I told her I could not handle another goodbye, but that didn't stop her from moving again.

She ended up moving to Washington to be closer to her son, so I wrote the color formula down for her to take to the new salon. She called me after her first hair appointment at the new place and wanted to make an appointment with me, since she didn't have a good experience. She drove four hours to get her hair done with me, and would sometimes stay for a night and drive back to Washington the next day. She said the lady didn't seem to know what she was doing, and she saw her use a color from a box you would get from the grocery store when you didn't know better. When I started doing her hair all those years ago, she would get so nervous and have me get a hand mirror for her so she could see what it looked like the minute the color was being washed off. I told her the color was hard to see when it was wet, since the water was in the hair cuticle, making it look darker. She lives in Eugene now, about an hour-and-a-half drive, but for her, it was worth it. We are going on thirty years together. We have been through raising our kids, celebrations and hardships, and shared so much. She is truly like family to me.

I tell my clients that it is team work, our relationship. They grow the hair, and I will maintain it, making it the best I can. For clients with brittle, over processed hair (brought on by themselves), I tell them to "dry clean only." Another client says she tell people it is her hair, but Debbie lets her wear it.

Another longtime client came in with flowers and told me it was his last haircut, that he was retiring and moving back to Texas. I really didn't think I heard him correctly, since I felt somewhat blindsided. I had cut his hair every four weeks for over twenty years. It would be a huge adjustment, and I would miss him. There was no warning, no time to prepare for his departure. As I cut his hair, we were both quiet, subdued in a way we were not accustomed to. He said he had been thinking about it all morning, how he had to say goodbye. As he went to leave, I told him to give me a hug. He picked me up off my feet, then set me down and left. I started crying as I watched him leave, and my next client was there, ready for his haircut. I had to excuse myself, go to the bathroom to calm myself down. It is hard when you have to turn off the waterworks sometimes. You try to think of a funny joke, and you think you have it under control, but the minute someone asks if you are all right, there they go again...more tears. The client who was waiting for me to get it together sat in my chair as I explained that my last client was moving away after cutting his hair for twenty years. This man had previously called and left a voice mail about how he didn't think he had forty-dollar hair. He was going to go somewhere else and thanked me for taking care of him. I was devastated. I felt at a loss, but the next day came another voice mail. He said he went out and got a haircut and, as it turned out, he does in fact have forty-dollar hair, and he asked if he could come in and have me fix it. I was elated to know he would be back.

When I greeted him, he bowed slightly and said, "I am sheepishly here to have you fix my hair."

After he saw me crying over the last client who was moving, I said, "You should have seen me after I got your message about going somewhere else. I sure missed you in that one day."

I was happy to get the phone call that my client would be back in town for a seminar. He could get a ride to the salon for his haircut, but he wasn't sure how he was going to get back to the hospital (this was pre-Uber days), so I offered him a ride. He then found out that he would be in town once a month for a year for these seminars, so we could schedule his haircut when he was in town, and he could put off looking for a new stylist to cut his hair in Texas. I would go and pick him up at the bus station, cut his hair, and then take him back to the bus station. I told him I had a cassette tape with my mom and I singing with Buck Owens that was recorded when I was six years old, and I told him I would play it for him the next time he was in town.

He said, "That's all right. You don't have to do that." I let him know I would love to share it with him. Again, he said I didn't have to do that. I then told him that he would have no choice than to listen to it, that he would be in my car, held hostage, and he'd be forced to listen to it. I think he thought I would forget all about it, but the next time I picked him up at the bus station, he got in my car, I hit the play button and there it was, six-year-old me, my mom, and Buck Owens singing, "I was looking back to see if you were looking back at me..." His quiet demeanor while listening to my tape made me turn it off and just enjoy his company. After the end of the year, when I dropped him off the last time, I had a sad moment on the drive back to the salon. It felt like an end of an era, and I wasn't sure he would ever sit in my chair again. We do email and stay in touch, but not on a regular basis. You really do miss your clients you have shared so much with over the years.

Years ago, when I was first starting out and was in a bad relationship, the kind that could affect your entire day, I read a passage saying that today was your gift. Do with it what you wanted, spend it how you wanted, and don't let anyone take it away from you. I was living this all one morning—didn't even let the driver who cut me off get to me. As I got to work, the receptionist told me she booked me with this older man, and she discreetly pointed him out to me under the desk, and then, with her hand by her head, signaled that she thought he was a bit crazy. I took it as my challenge to see if I would still stay in my chipper mood, not letting anything or anyone get me down. I walked over to the man, calling him by name, telling him my name, and had him follow me to my station where we could begin our conversation.

He kept saying, "I want a perm. Just don't louse it up!" I tried talking to him about his past perms and what he was looking for, and again, he mentioned not to louse it up.

After his repeated abuse to me, I turned to him and told him, "If you think I am going to louse up your hair, you can go somewhere else. I am in a good mood today, and I am not going to let you ruin it."

He just looked at me, sort of surprised and said, "You know, you're all right." He liked that I stood up for myself. As I earned his trust, he came back to me again and again. Turned out, he was just upset with the world after losing his wife to cancer. He would say the grumpiest things, putting him in the grumpy old man club. You know you've met a grumpy old man when he uses the phrase, "Oh for crap's sake!" Then one day, I was running ten minutes late for him, and he stormed out, and I never saw him again.

I feel bad if I am late for some reason. Chances are I am late because the prior client was late. I try to stay on time, and if I know I will be late, I will text the next client and give him or her a heads up. One time, I did just that, letting the client know I would be fifteen minutes late. He used to just come back to my station, somehow getting past the warden (the receptionist) and stand with his arms folded, looking at me as if it was his time.

His posture said, "Why is someone else in my chair?" It was uncomfortable, and I felt rushed. He really gave it to me this one day for being late after I called to say I would be. I mentioned I called him to let him know, and he said he should get a discount since I was not on time. I was not the pizza place where it was free if it took more than thirty minutes to deliver. Besides, he did autopsies for a living. I wanted to ask him if he was keeping his patients waiting, but I thought better of it.

TAKING YOUR WORK
HOME WITH YOU

I do take my work home with me. I am usually covered with little hair shavings at the end of the day. The first thing you do when you get home is de-hair. If I am still at work and having lunch, sometimes there will be a cut hair in my food. It really doesn't faze you when you have had it happen for years. Usually, you just take it out and think, "There's Bob's hair." It is not that bad, unless it is a long hair with that bulb on the end, and you wonder who's scalp it came from—then I am grossed out.

The hair really sticks to you. You find it in all sorts of places you would never dream it would go. The hairs on the chest are the most popular. Maybe since I lotion up in the morning, it attracts the hair and keeps it there. Sometimes, you have to get the tweezers out and do surgery. They work their way into your nipple, or somehow get stuck between your teeth and gums. I guess I shouldn't laugh so much; seems I'm inhaling them in. I was clothes shopping once, and as I was perusing the little boutique, the sales lady asked me if I liked a sweater she was holding in my view. I told her I try to stay away from sweaters since I do hair for a living, and the cut hair slivers embed in the knit. She told me her mom used to do hair, and she remembered her pulling out a three-inch hair from her nipple.

I just smiled and shook my head. "Yes, it happens," is all I said.

In the summertime, if you wear sandals, they can get embedded in the bottom of your foot, and you will have to operate to free the hair slivers. One day, I knew I had a hair in the bottom of my foot, but could not see it. I looked for it over and over throughout the week. It was so sore, and I couldn't put my full weight on my foot since it was so bothersome. When I came home at the end of my week, I had to just dig that hair out, knowing I would have a couple of days to recover. I got a needle out and just kept digging until I found it. It was a white, strong hair. No wonder I couldn't see it. Sometimes, you can look at the bottom of your foot and see a few hairs that are working their way in, but haven't completed their job. That's when I get the tape roller out and go to town.

I once lost a toenail to a cut hair. During tap class, I wore a new pair of tap shoes that needed breaking in. After class, as I took off the shoes and viewed the damage I was feeling to my feet, I saw I was left with a blister on my big toe. Eventually, the blister popped, and a cut hair worked its way in there, under my toenail. It festered up enough to make me schedule an appointment with my doctor. She ended up having to cut my toenail off, which was not a good feeling. First, she wrapped a rubber band around my toe, taking the edge off a little, so she said, enough to dispense a shot to numb it the rest of the way. Then she started cutting the nail off. Meanwhile, I was about to pass out, and I wanted to know which client of mine this cut hair belonged to. He or she was going to pay! I told a few of my clients it was their hair that was found under there and they believed me. I guessed I had a trusting face.

The strange thing was, while at the grocery store, there was this strange guy following me around, giving me that interested look that I was not giving it back. I was ready to say I was involved if he asked me out. Even if you are not in a relationship, you can still say you are involved and they think you are involved with another guy. It is not a lie. You are involved with shopping and breathing. You don't have to get involved with your involvement. It really works. You can even say it as if you are a bit disappointed that you are involved. They move right along. I have shared this bit of information with my single female clients, telling them how I have used it on occasions. One of my clients reported back to me, telling me how it worked for her.

This guy was behind me in the checkout line, and I could feel him checking me out. I could almost feel his breath on my neck, he was standing so close, so I turned to face him, hoping he would get the hint and back away. He just looked at me, so I turned around in search of an open checker ready to ring my items. Then I felt his grip on my big toe. I looked down, and he actually had my toe in his grasp. Who touches a toe? Just randomly? I extracted my toe from his grip, and he asked me if I just had my toes done.

I said, "No," and then heard him say, "I want you." Finally, the checker motioned he was free, so I darted away from the foot fetish guy, paid, and then ran to my car, not wanting another encounter in the parking lot. Soon after, my toe was acting up, so I joked that the strange guy in the grocery store who grabbed my toe put a hex on it. Really, it was just a cut hair that had gone into the popped blister opening, causing an infection, leading to the dismissal of a toe worth grabbing. That was when I decided I was living on the edge with such a dangerous profession.

Sometimes, while standing behind another customer at the grocery store checkout line, I will look at hair and say to myself, "Judging by this guy's hairline, he had a haircut nine days ago." I'm always so curious and almost want to ask. I did ask a lady one day if she had just gotten a haircut. She had! I just told her I was a hair stylist, so that was how I knew, but really, she had cut hairs all over her shoulders. It made me take note to always clean my clients off. Other times, I would study the lady's hair in front of me in the checkout line, deciding what colors were used for her hair color, or think how a 9.32 would really add a nice tone to her hair. I cannot turn this off. It is something I feel I could do in my sleep.

I tell this to clients and, sometimes, during a cut, I will say, "See?" and then close my eyes while cutting.

I take more than hair home with me. Sometimes, throughout the day, I will hear good stories from my clients. One client was telling me how she could not find her glasses and that she needed to find them fast, so she could see. She had a mishap in the shower at a prestigious health club. She said she was in the shower and she spotted something on the floor, so she picked it up. As she brought it closer to her face, she said it was round and brown and that it was a turd! I could not continue cutting her hair because I was in hysterics.

She followed with, "Some biddy didn't just drop it! It didn't just fall out!"

I asked, "Did you drop it, or throw it?'" She said she walked it over to the garbage. Knowing her, she seemed to speak her mind, writing letters to organizations she did not agree with. I asked her if she reported it. Now I could just see her marching up to the front desk, reporting such an incident of how she could barely see and was doing her part by helping clean up garbage on the shower floor, but she discovered it was a turd. I awaited the answer I already knew.

"Yes," she said, and I couldn't control myself. This was the funniest thing I thought I had ever heard; I had to wipe my tears.

Whenever this client comes in, we end up laughing so hard, we're snorting, which makes us laugh harder. She had a little fight with her neighbor and said she left a note for her on her garbage can. I sometimes drive past her house since it was near where I pick my daughter up after work. One night after she was in, as I drove by, I looked at the garbage can, and there was her note posted. Now, over the next four years, I would have so much material on her complaints that I would have another chapter. I have told her about this book I have been writing, fourteen-plus years in the making, and will tell her a few of my stories, and she tells me she is going home to write my book.

THE KITCHEN CUT

When I was first starting out, I did a lot of haircutting in the kitchen. I had a few monthly-paid haircuts, since some of them didn't want to go to the beauty school and have the instructor "recut" their hair, and they thought they were doing me a favor. I wouldn't have to split the entire nine dollars with anyone else, a quid pro quo. I got to keep it all for myself. Wow! I wasn't fond of the kitchen cut because I was always worried about getting hair all over, since I am a clean freak. I would try to contain the hair, keeping it in the perimeters, close to the person I was cutting, sort of compartmentalizing it away from the cooking elements. I would hate to be cooking dinner and discover a cut hair in the salad. That would be enough to shut the kitchen cuts down, at least until I was established.

Sometimes, I would do a few cuts at a time. Might as well, since I already had the mess and was in haircutting mode. Nothing like making a few extra bucks doing something I loved, on a day off. But as I got busier at work, the kitchen cuts were losing their charm. They started interloping on my free time, and I had to put an end to them.

Have Shears Will Travel

I do make house calls, not that I advertise for that. I have clients that I have cut for over twenty years, which I refer to as the twenty-year club, and I will drive to them and make house calls when necessary. There was an older couple I saw for many years. I cut the woman's hair for over twenty years and knew her husband since he would drive her to see me, and when it was almost time for her to be finished, I would call him to give him the fifteen-minute pick-up time. As they got to be in their nineties, he could no longer drive her, so I would go to them and cut their hair in their kitchen. When she needed a perm, since it was too hard of a task for the kitchen, I would pick her up and take her to the salon, then take her home and cut her husband's hair. One time, while driving home, we were at a red light. She looked over and saw a sign that said BRAZILIAN WAXING. She asked if it was a Brazilian grocery store.

I said, "No, they do waxing."

"Like bikini waxing?" she asked.

"Sort of," I said, "But there, they do the whole thing. All of the hair...gone." And I made a little hand gesture as if I was backhand swatting a fly, whistling at the same time, for the effect.

"Oh," she said. "Some things just need hair. They're not very attractive." I had to turn my head to discreetly laugh out the driver side window. The cute thing about this lady was that I could just see her going home, and after I left, she would share with her husband about the Brazilian store that she saw—actually waxing everything clean—and his response would be, "Oh my."

One day, as I was driving her to the salon on perm day, it was raining so hard.

She said, "Oh my! It is raining so hard, we can barely see. We should pull over and wait until it lets up." Well, I had five hours ahead of me to perm her hair and cut her husband's hair in the kitchen, so I had to reassure her that I could see, and trudged along. She wouldn't let me take the freeway, since it scared her, even though I would reassure her I was an excellent driver.

I went over to their house on her ninety-first birthday to take her some cake, and she asked me to help her make her bed. As I was on the side I was making, she asked me how far the covers were hanging down, and I gave her a rough estimate. She was very precise and wanted both sides exactly the same. It was taking so long to make the bed, and it felt as if it was at least eighty-six degrees in there; I had to take off my jacket. She had to walk over to my side to see how much was hanging over. It took thirty-five minutes to make the bed. I wondered how long it would have taken her if I had not been there to help. I always wanted to help. As I would drop her off after a haircut, she would have little duties for me to do.

She would say, "I was going to stand on a chair and do it." I did not want her to ever have to stand on a chair. So I would clean the dining room light and get the cob webs up high in the corners. I helped her wind up her outside awning, and it was as tight as I could get it, but she always had to "check" to see if it was as tight as it could go. She had these clocks that were from the 1800s that needed winding. I would get the key and wind them, I guess too fast for her liking, but I am quick that way. She was always so worried I would break them. I would say, "I won't break them. I'm just a fast winder." I would just shake my head and laugh, hoping that one day, what goes around comes around, and I would have some young hair stylist to help me with looking good and household tasks if I threatened to get a chair to stand on.

She always wanted me to park in her garage. When it was time for me to show up there, she would have the garage door opened for me. One day, I was supposed to be there at five o'clock, after working a full day. I pulled into the driveway, and the garage door was closed. I called her, and she said I was early, that she was just getting out of the shower. I waited for a bit, and then she opened the door. She was standing there in the doorway with a hand towel draped in front of her naked body. As I entered the house, she turned and walked into the bathroom. I shook my head, and looked away from her backside.

"Oh boy," I said to myself. "I didn't need to see that." Since she had kitchen carpet, I had to get a plastic shower liner I had purchased to put down, and it was kept in the garage. After each haircut, I would have to take my cape out to the front yard to shake all of the lose hair out before I would blow-dry, so I would not scatter it all over the kitchen. I would always wet my finger and hold it up to check the direction of the wind, so the hair would not end up all over me.

I would set up shop and wait. When she was dressed and ready for her cut, she told me she wanted me to park in the garage. I told her I had already turned my car off, since the door was closed when I arrived, and it was just sixteen feet away from the garage, but no, she wanted me in the garage. I went back out to move my car. She was very high maintenance, but I loved her and felt so close to her. That was the last time I saw her. She had me rub medicine on her back shingles, and I was thinking how this was not part of my job description, that she needed a caregiver to help her. I have comfort in knowing she thought of me as family, and we did have so many nice years together. Sometimes, though, after doing way more than I had planned on—since I usually had to go back to work—and she stood there waving goodbye to me, I would seat belt in, put it in reverse, and as I was backing out of the driveway, I would wave and say to myself, "I'm so getting into heaven."

One time, I was talked into driving to nowhere land to do a cut on my kid's uncle. "Oh, it is not that far from where you are," he said. I was out of town visiting my mom and aunt on Memorial Day weekend. Before I agreed to this, I asked him if there was a place for him to sit for me to do a proper haircut. I knew he had cattle and pictured myself cutting in the barn. Something to add

187

to my "places I have cut hair" repertoire. I ended up driving over two hours to get there, when I was told it would take thirty-five minutes. There were huge potholes in the road that my bug could not handle. By the time I got there, I saw his truck parked along the shoulder of the dirt road. There was no place to cut his hair but on a tailgate, and I was too classy for that, so I was livid! I saw him down in the canyon, burning brush. I yelled, "It took me over two hours to get here and there is no place to cut your hair!" I swore I heard my echo. I was so mad. I ended up pulling out my zebra cape and cut his hair along the side of the road as he sat on a bucket. I had only my spray bottle to wet down his smoky, sweaty hair. The wind was blowing and with each cut, it would blow the hair back onto me. It was so surreal. I couldn't believe I had gone back so far, as if I were just starting out, cutting hair in the yard. I mean, I did not have to do that anymore! I was a seasoned hair stylist and felt disrespected. I just wanted to go out of town for the weekend to visit my family and was talked into going to the country to do a haircut on the uncle since he could not make it to town. I wanted to drive home another way, but ended up going out of my way for that. It was very upsetting, and there was no place to wash my hands. I got home late that night and couldn't believe I did a country cut!

One of my clients was growing his hair out. He had this idea to move to Hawaii, and since I would not be there to cut his hair, he said he might as well have a ponytail so he would not need my services. I had cut his hair for twenty-five years, and he could not imagine anyone else cutting it. The growing out stages were bad, and his hair was very thick. One day, he came in with it piled down, covering his ears.

As we were talking, he kept saying, "What?" He couldn't hear.

I said, "Well there is no wonder you can't hear me, with that hair muff you have over your ears. If it is affecting your hearing, you should get rid of it." Then the day came, and there was finally enough hair to gather in a small ponytail. Seemed after that, I never saw him, since he was wearing the low-maintenance hair and was trying to wean off my services. One day, I got a panicked call from him, saying how he woke up in the morning, went to the bathroom, and looked in the mirror and had to blink a few times to make it register if he was really seeing what he thought he was seeing. His ponytail was gone. He looked down by the floor, and a bucket was there where his ponytail was lying. I asked him what happened, and he said his girlfriend must have cut his hair while he was sleeping.

He had to come in so I could fix the wreckage that was left on his head. What kind of girlfriend cuts her boyfriend's hair while he lay sleeping? He ended up not moving to Hawaii and broke up with his girlfriend. It would be hard to stay with someone after that person defiled your hair. I mean, twenty-five years without a hair affair, and then you fall asleep one night and wake with a new hairdo. That is grounds for a break up. Otherwise you would always have to hide all sharp implements before you turn out the lights at night, or sleep with one eye open.

One of my clients was battling cancer. As she was losing her hair, she was unsure of what to do. She thought it best to come to the salon to have me cut it all off. She was a very special client to me. I told her I would go to her house to cut it in private. I thought it would make her feel better, not having other clients around, wondering what was going on with her. As I arrived at her house, I was thankful her daughter was there as well. I knew it would be a hard task to do. She loved her hair and would come in on special occasions just to have it styled. As I got the clippers out, I could not face her, for fear she would see the tears in my eyes. I wanted to be strong for her. When it was all done, and her hair lay in a pile on the floor, she went to the bathroom to look in the mirror. I was not sure what to expect of her reaction. She came out with a smile on her face and thanked me. Her daughter was teasing her that she looked like Gollum from *The Lord of the Rings*. She then crouched down on the floor and started mimicking him. We all started laughing, and it ended up lightening the mood and being a fun day that I would never forget. She ended up losing her life to cancer. She touched my life in a way that I will always hold dear, and I have a special place in my heart for her—for Patty.

I have another lady I pick up and take home after I have cut her hair. I call it Driving Miss Daisy. Usually, she wants to go to Kentucky Fried Chicken on the way home, which is fine with me.

As I am going through the drive-through, ordering what I was instructed to order, she would yell, in her New York accent, "Make sure I get cold slawer! Are you going to throw in a biscuit?" She had ordered the meal, so I reassured her she would get the biscuit; besides, we were no longer near the ordering menu, out of the two-way speaker zone, closer to the person who was in the little takeout window. She then asked him again about the biscuit. I just sat there and smiled to myself. All I could think was, *I hope she doesn't get home and they forgot her biscuit.* Other times, she had a few more stops to make. She didn't drive herself, so I would drive Miss Daisy. I had to help her draw her right leg into my car, then seat belt her in. So every time she has an errand to run after her haircut, we go through this process. I try to make it quick, but it is not a fast task, and she tells me she has to go to the bank, or I will not get paid. When she gets out of my car, she rocks and counts to three before she tries to get out. Some of our conversations are hilarious.

Once, the moment she got in my car, she started talking, and I was driving, saying, "Uh-huh."

She said, "I had a rash under my breasts. As you get older, your boobs sag, so after the shower you have to use a talc, and I used a talc, and I still got a rash."

I muttered, "Uh-huh."

"I went to pick out underwear and they were out of my size eight. Oh, you don't think I wear size eight," she said.

I had to say more. "I believe you wear size eight."

I went to a convalescent home to cut a client's hair one hot July day, and the air conditioning was on the fritz, so it was stiflingly hot in the room. Her roommate was getting her diaper changed, so it was hot and unpleasant. As I waited for my client to come out of the bathroom so I could begin my job, I was trying to stay focused. As I cut her hair, I heard the bathroom door close, and it occurred to me that another resident who was on the other side of the bathroom was occupying the adjoined facility. I could hear the person in there, making the most disgusting bodily sounds, and I was trying to tune him or her out. After the haircut, my client went back into the bathroom to brush her teeth before dinner. Her daughter went out to her car to get a check to pay me for my services, so I watched my client in case she needed my help. I saw her spot the mess in the toilet, and she grabbed a couple of squares of toilet paper and put her hand in the toilet to clean the leftover splatter.

I yelled for her daughter, saying, "Your mom has her hand in the toilet bowl!" She told her mom to get her hand out of the toilet.

The mom replied, "I was trying to clean it!" As she started to brush her teeth, she didn't recognize her toothbrush, and I heard her say, "Hey! This is not my toothbrush!" I ran to tell the daughter about the toothbrush, and she came in to tell her mom it was her new one. By the time I left, I felt traumatized, since I was type A. It made me think of how that could be me years from now, and maybe I would not have all of my faculties and would want to clean up the mess in the toilet and not recognize my toothbrush. I think the heat was getting to me that day, but I did leave feeling a little down. It was sad to see your clients in that state.

I went to another convalescent home to cut one of my older client's hair. She was so happy to see me, and after I fixed her all up, I rolled her around in the wheel chair as she gave me the tour. One of the male nurses commented on her hair, saying how nice it looked.

She said, "This is my hairdresser. She fixed me up," as she patted me on the hand. It gave me such joy, seeing her so happy. There are so many of my clients who are special to me. It is my job to do their hair, but to me, it isn't just a job. I love what I do, but I love it more when I can help someone out who is in need, to make people feel better and brighten their days, because it also brightens my day, and that is the most fulfilling part for me.

THE BRUSH AND THE MUSTACHE COMB

I had a male client who had gone to the same stylist for over thirty years. When his stylist retired, I was lucky and got him. We had always talked while he was in, and I felt as if I knew him. I had watched him in the mirror for years since my station was directly behind where he sat for his previous haircuts. When the time would come, the final comb, he would stand close to the mirror, find his part, and comb his hair to his liking. He wouldn't just comb and part; he would study it in the mirror, comb it forward to get the part just so. I used to tease him.

When he sat in my chair for the first haircut, and it came time to style, I told him he could stand and look in the mirror up close to get his part. He was shocked that I knew his parting routine. See, I did know what was going on at the other stations around me. I paid attention, which I thought impressed him a little.

He stood to part his hair but struggled. It seemed to me that when someone has a serious part such as his, it would be trained to just fall into place with just a snap of the fingers. I started to sweat a bit, thinking I did not live up to the haircut he had been used to getting for over thirty years. He told me he used a special brush. I asked him about this brush and the special powers it had over his part and if he had it with him. He did. It was in his car. He carried it with him wherever he went. I told him to go get it and bring it in. I was expecting this brush to be carried in a special case, or that it was gold plated, but it was a normal-looking brush. I called it the woody goody, since it is a goody brush, made out of that fake wood, such as the kind on the *Brady Bunch* station wagon. I thought it would send off a ray of light, the way he talked about it, but it was even missing a section of bristles. Turned out, he had five other brushes like it. One at home, one at the office, car, gym bag, et cetera. I asked him to leave it with me, so when he came in, he could find his part. Sometimes, I stepped away and gave him alone time with his brush to find his part, or I swept and did my own thing, giving him ample time to comb it in place.

He always had a routine he ran through while in the chair. When I cut his ear hair, I noticed one hair was way back in the folds of the ear. It liked to hide, and I pretended I was a single ear hair that was up against the wall, standing still, not wanting to be spotted. He asked me about that hair and if it was hiding, and he made the face I made when I pretended to be the hair.

Also, he asked, "How's my brow?" I studied it, noticed he had gone to town on it, and I did the best I could. In the end, I rinsed all of the cut hairs out of his hair, and he always said, "Hose me down and put me away wet." We always laughed a lot. He is a fun client to look forward to. It is hard, though, after cutting his hair, laughing as much as we do, to get a more sedated client who just wants to relax. I start to get the giggles thinking about some of the things we laughed about, and I have to really keep myself in the moment and just be on auto pilot and cut. You really have to mold to your clients' personalities. After all, it is their time, and if they want to be quiet, you should be quiet. His wife comes in to see me as well, so it is a hair party in my studio with the two of them. We get to laughing so hard sometimes, it is hard to remember I have a job to do. I look forward to their visits, and it makes my job feel as though it isn't a job at all. Like we are at a party, having the time of our lives.

So now, when he comes in, I always have his brush out and ready for him. Sometimes, I put a candy on it, such as a chocolate kiss. One time, I cut out of the paper a picture of Cheryl Burke from *Dancing with the Stars* and taped it to his brush, since that was his favorite dancer. We always have fun, and then he combs his hair one last time and says goodbye to his brush. Thank goodness every client doesn't have a special brush. I don't know where I would store them all.

When I moved to a new salon, I told him how I was going to carry his brush out special, pack it in bubble wrap, and place it on my dash, not just throw it in with the rest of them, for his woody goody missing bristles is a special brush with special parting powers.

I have another guy who had me trim his beard and mustache. I did the best I could, but everyone has their own version of what their mustache should look like. They know how they like it, and the certain angle they are used to it having. Everyone wears it differently. One of my clients brought in a little mustache comb in a snack-size ziplock baggy. He thought it would aid in achieving the line he liked. It did work wonders and allowed me to cut it the way he preferred. So now, in my drawer of brushes, I have the woody goody and the little mustache comb.

THE COUGAR

I had a new client in, and upon my first impression, I had no idea she would turn out to be such a cougar. She told me she was eighty-seven and that she was dating a younger man.

I asked her how old the younger man was, and she replied, "eighty-one." I told her she was a cougar and explained that was when an older woman dated a younger man. "Oh," she said. "I am a cougar." I told her that cougars pounce on their prey, and she said, "Oh, I pounce!" It was so funny coming from her since she looked like a sweet, innocent grandma. She went on to tell me about her date with this younger man and how he took her to the Red Lobster. When they got in the car after the meal, she pounced on him to give him a kiss and knocked his glasses off.

He'd said, "We better get out of here before we're arrested."

She came in one day and told me she told her man she was a cougar. He asked what it was and how she knew about it. She told him it was an older woman and a younger man, and that she read a lot. Sometimes, you just cannot help but laugh out loud. You have to take a breather, even if you were in mid-haircutting or using the blow-dryer, to just stop and laugh. Sometimes, I snort, and then that really gets things going.

I started teasing her about being a cougar when she would come in weekly to have me style her hair for her younger man. She said that her neighbor noticed she had a new hairdo, complimenting her from across the street. It was fun when she came in, and I looked forward to teasing her about her younger man.

I called my cougar client one time to get her in for an appointment, and she said she was exercising in bed.

I asked, "Do you mind me asking, are you alone?" She said she was alone and was just stretching, that she wasn't doing the mattress mambo. She said it was a good thing her boyfriend had erectile dysfunction, otherwise they would be rolling around in bed for hours.

One time, she wanted a shorter, sassy haircut, but she had thinning hair on the top where her scalp was exposed. I told her I would leave it longer on the top to hide the thinning spot and perk up the rest. As I was cutting the neckline shorter, she must have thought I was cutting her bald. She told me that if I cut too much hair, she was going to take my shears and cut a chunk of hair out of my head and paste it on her head! I knew she wouldn't do that, but the visual sent me into hysterics again and made me aware of the whereabouts of my shears. When I finished styling, I showed her how cute and sassy she was. I then mentioned that I couldn't believe she said she would cut my hair if she didn't like it. She told me she was looking at a nice thick piece of my hair in the back that she would like to have. I thought I would hide my shears from now on and not leave them out in the open, up for grabs, or not turn my back to her.

I just loved when she came in, and I can only hope to be like her one day, having such a zest for life. She had been through so much in her life but choose to be happy. She told me she put on some black underwear and a lacy bra and walked out to show her boyfriend.

She asked him, "So what do you think of an eighty-seven-year-old woman in black underwear?"

He said, "Come a little closer. I can't see."

She would tell me how she was planning to wear a nice lacy bra to the theater and wished she could show it off, but then she said, "At least I will know I have it on."

I asked her if she had confessed her love to this younger man. She had not been brave enough to tell him she loved him. I was telling her that if she lipped the words "Olive juice," it would look as if she were saying, "I love you." This way, she didn't have to be nervous about rejection. If he didn't respond, she can always point out she didn't say those words, that she just had a love for olive juice. She did this in the mirror a few times and then licked her lips back and forth quickly, with her best sultry face. I asked what she was doing, and she told me she was trying to be sexy. I told her it looked as if she were licking butter from her lips and that she should do it slower, just once, corner to corner, as I would know.

She did it again and said, "I've done that before when I licked across a man's body." I never knew what she would say and am reminded to enjoy the moment.

One time, as I was putting her purse on my counter and she was about to sit in my chair, she told me I had a cute bottom. What do you say to that? Thank you.

She said, "Well you do. I got a good look." Another time, as I was helping her zip her coat, I was bent over enough, and she said, "I like that," and pointed to what I thought was my necklace. I touched my necklace, remembering which one I was wearing to tell her where it had come from, and she said, "No. I like those." I then realized she was pointing to my slightly exposed cleavage. She told me she liked what she saw and thought I should bend over just a little when my boyfriend was over to give him a little show. Another stylist close by heard what she was saying and just started laughing. She was quite the cougar, and I wouldn't have wanted her to be any other way.

She would drive herself to the salon, which was close to her house, but hard to get out of. When it was time for her to leave, I would go out and get her car ready, point it in the direction of her home and walk her out. Then the day came when her boyfriend passed away. He was not doing so well, and as she sat in my chair, telling me about it, she had one single tear on her cheek the entire time. It was so sad.

Her daughter-in-law would drive her to see me for her haircuts, as it was getting harder for her to drive. I always enjoyed my time with her. She was a real mood brightener. She called me her little movie star hairdresser. She is now gone, but I will treasure my time with her and remind myself that life is short. She taught me you need to have fun and spread sunshine along the way, while wearing a lacy bra.

TO BEND OR NOT TO BEND

Some clients have benders, some don't. You are cutting the clients' hair, and you need to get the hair that is behind the ear, which is a hard area to get, since the ear is totally in your way. You go to fold the ear forward, but it will not bend. It doesn't matter how many times you try; the ear is not going anywhere. It is as if it's on steroids and besides that, it's inflexible. You think to yourself, *They must have more cartilage than most people.* You try to just comb the hair down in front of the ear, but you still cannot get an even line. You go to the other side of the head to the other ear to see if it will cooperate, but they are in cahoots, as if they are in an alliance to stand their ground. You note to yourself that this client does not have benders. You can try to push it out of your way, fold it forward, but it will not budge. You do the best you can, trying to get a clean line around the ear, and move on.

Back in beauty school, when I was working on the floor and finished with a haircut, I had to have the instructor come and inspect it. One time, I thought I did a perfect haircut, but then the instructor bent the client's ear down, folded it down flush, and really got behind the ear, giving the cut a cleaner line with less bulk behind the ear. That was impressive to me since I was OCD and wanted the hair to lay just right. I had never done that before. The mannequins we had to work on in class did not have real ear parts that we could maneuver out of the way. They had a hairline, but not a single ear for you to practice moving. I would always remember that method, and it was how I can tell a good haircut, when the hair was not a long strip that was left, since the ear was a bender.

The first time I bent an ear to cut the hair that hid stubbornly behind it was when I was still in beauty school and doing kitchen cuts. I was too embarrassed to bend his ear forward. I was shy back then, and it seemed way too personal of a task. I had my roommate bend his ear while I cut the hair. I have seen stylists who get their clients to hold their own ears while cutting in the ear zone. It makes since when using the clippers. You don't always have an extra hand for ear holding. For those of you who know me, I am totally opposite now, not shy about moving ears. I could handle ears all day.

There should be an ear exercise for those ears that don't bend. You know you have a haircut coming up. You could try bending them, doing three sets of eight a few times a night—get them relaxed enough to bend to get a cleaner line.

THE OUT-OF-TOWNERS

I have clients who have a ton of hair. I told one guy that I was tired just thinking about cutting his hair, since he had so much. He knew who he was. I booked out extra time for him, since he was so well endowed in the hair department. Plus, he was the furthest traveled client. He moved to Virginia sixteen years ago and still came in for haircuts. He would text me, set up his haircut day and time, and fly into town. If he had to miss a haircut appointment with me, he would email me to tell me about the affair. He was open about it; there was no shame, only regret.

In his email, it was usually a funny story of how the stylist did or did not do what I normally did. He had even sent a picture of his bad haircut. Attached would be a file that I would open, and there he would be, head tilted, with a funny look on his face as if he was trying to tell me his hair was unhappy. I thought this made him appreciate me more. He mentioned how he was the furthest traveled client and wanted to come in to see a plaque on my wall with his name. So I made a corny sign out of cardboard and put his name on there and displayed it before I brought him back to my station.

He had so much hair that I liked to make up little songs to sing to him. I liked to pretend I could rap. "You have the biggest hair, but I don't care, when I'm done, I'll charge you double fare." One day, I was running an errand before his appointment time, and I got a flat tire. I had to take it to Les Schwab to get new ones, so I had to reschedule him. This was when he lived in town. Had he lived out of town, traveling that far, I would have done everything to make it back to cut his hair. I felt I owed him an apology song.

Thank goodness it went to voice mail, as I sang, "I'm so sorry, I missed your hair. I didn't want you to think I didn't care. My tire was flat, so I used my spare, went to Les Schwab and got a brand-new pair."

When he was in need of a haircut, he called it an "advanced." My business cards at the time said ADVANCED HAIRCUTTING. I used to call to tell him the day before he came in that I would rest my hands for his upcoming cut, and that I would wear oven mitts on my hands to protect them to get ready for the *advanced*. I also had a client from Alaska, but she moved back to town. Now she could come in for bang trims and not have to attend the bang trimmers support group.

I do not charge more for clients who have more hair. I should, though. I charge less if they have less hair. Maybe I should just have one fee, and if I get someone who has a lot of hair and another who has less, it will just be a wash.

For clients who have a ton of hair, I love to say things such as, "I really have my work cut out for me." Or, "I am tired just thinking about cutting your hair." The best, "I don't think I have even put a dent in your hair yet." I love to play it up—act like I am so exhausted. Actually, when blow-drying someone with a lot of hair, I do get a tired arm and just have to put my arms down for a second, maybe take a drink of water, and tell them they have a one ton bun. I also point out the workout they can get from blow-drying their own hair in the morning, hoping if I ever run into them out in public, it would be what I always pictured it would be as the client walked out of the salon door.

It is funny when you run into clients outside of the salon. Some of them act as if they don't want to see you. One lady was acting strange, saying she was in a hurry, and the next time she came in for her appointment, she confessed that she had cut her bangs that we were trying to grow out and didn't want me to see them. I didn't notice that day, since she had her new baby with her. I wasn't paying attention to her hair. Another client I ran into told me not to look at her hair, that she didn't have time to fix it before she left. I wondered how many of my clients were walking around, not styled. It's like people's children: the last time you see them is the age you always picture them when you think of them, even though ten years have gone by. The same is true with my clients. The last time I see them, after I have fixed them up, that is how their hair looks in my mind, until I see them again. I was behind a lady in line, and I recognized the back of her head. I said her name, and she turned around. I just knew it was her. I stand there, behind my clients, looking at the back of their heads. I could spot them anywhere.

I had a young man who was in high school who would come in for his quarterly haircuts. He would only come in every four months. Sometimes, in longer spans. His hair was always so big and full. It was a curly afro.

He would come in and say, "Today, the fro must go."

I would know how much to cut off, know just where to take it down to, and I would even say, "Let's take this down a notch." He told me the only thing he didn't like, when his hair was short, was that his bubble space was gone. People stood back when he had the fro and got closer to him, invading his personal space, when it was shorter. I could agree with him. I could see standing back from a fro. You never knew what was going to be hidden in there.

We liked to experiment with his hair, although, there was only one cut that worked with his hair. One day, we tried to give him a faux hawk. I sectioned off the top of the hair that I wanted to keep longer, cutting the other hair short. The moment I released the top hair from the clip, it spread out over the entire top of his head, like a puff ball had just been set there. I tried taking more out of that section, just leaving a small amount to make the faux hawk, but it didn't matter how little the section was; it was not going to perform. He then called it a "fro hawk." Sometimes he will wear these creations out and enjoy them for a few days and come back to have the rest taken off. He has great hair, so we might as well have fun with it.

He had the idea of doing the reverse rat tail. Seemed he could talk me into these things, even though it was against my better judgment. We left a little piece out in the front to see how long it could grow. You couldn't tell it was there, since his hair was so curly; he could just tuck it into the rest of his hair, and it would stay hidden.

THE ONLY ONE

S ome clients think they are your only client. Maybe that is why they are late. They don't think you have anyone else coming in after them, so they can do as they please, be on their own schedule. I have a client who is always early. He comes and peeks around the corner to spy on me. He always makes a comment about the prior client who was sitting in "his" chair, as if he is the only one. I reassure him that I have a lot more clients, even open the client card box, thumb from A to Z, and let him get a good look. He is not the only one, and if he is not careful, he will be the only one getting the boot!

Knowing he is waiting, I take my time, sweep and clean, bus my station, and tell him that he is early and that I am not on the clock yet, to just chill. He waits in the shampoo room and relaxes in the bowl. While shampooing him, I have the sudden urge to use cold water. Just the thought makes me smile, and I am ready to do his hair. Sometimes, it's the little naughty thoughts about doing something that fulfill an impulse internally, so you don't have to act on it. Now that I am working in my studio, and I can close and lock my door, I find myself doing this before he comes in. When I am really busy, and need to have a minute to eat, I will lock my door.

One time, I had just locked my door and sat back down to finish eating when he tried to open it, saying, "Open the door." I was so pleased with myself for locking it when I did.

I just calmly said, "Have a seat in the hall. You're early, I'm finishing my lunch in peace, and I'm not on the clock yet." If I really want to drive my point across, I also close my curtain. That is the only thing about my work place—not having a receptionist to greet them and let them know I will be out when I can, so the clients will sit on a chair in the hall and stare in at you and your client, as if they are at the zoo and you are the monkey behind the glass.

The most often asked question is, "Am I your last client?" Even if it is noon, they still ask. Do you know why? They want to be, because they want to leave thinking that they are your only client: the most special one, but if that were the case, how would I be able to support my family? If they were my only client, I would question why no one else was coming in to see me. Was I that bad that I could not get any more clients? I couldn't afford to be in the business, and they would be forced to sit in another chair asking about their clientele. I do treat my clients as if they are my only ones. I want them to have my undivided attention, to feel relaxed and not rushed, as if I am rushing to the next thirty-eight clients of the day.

One of my clients asked if he was one of my favorites. How did I respond to that question?

My mind said, "Not really," but what came out of my mouth was, "Well, I have so many other clients I've had longer who are in front of you."

He said, "Where am I on the ladder?"

I asked, "What type of ladder are we talking about? If it is a step ladder, then you are not even in the garage, but if it is a big ladder, the one you use to reach high places, you may be in line to get on the first step."

He said, "I am not even on the bottom rung?" Recently, we celebrated our seven-year hairiversary. He said he hoped he had climbed a few rungs, that it had been seven years of "hairtal bliss," and for that, I decided to make room for him on the bottom rung.

I have so many longtime clients I like to celebrate with when it is our hair anniversary, which I call the hairiversary. I have a lot of twenty-year and twenty-five-year clients and one thirty-year client. I've taken some to dinner, happy hour, or breakfast. One man had been in my chair for twenty-five years, so we met for breakfast to celebrate. The first time he was in, I asked him how he was referred to me.

He said, "You held open the door for my wife at the salon. She asked who you were and then set up an appointment for me to come in." When I first met him, he asked me where I was from.

I told him, "A little town in eastern Oregon that you probably haven't heard of called Burns."

He said, "Heard of it. I was born there." I didn't believe him at first, but it ended up being the truth, and it was a match made in heaven right there. He was fifty-six when he started coming to me. Now, he's eighty-three, and he's the sweetest man. I look forward to more celebrations with him.

A guy client came in one day and was joking about getting a Mohawk. I started cutting his hair as I always did, knowing that one, he was too old for such a hairdo; two, he didn't ride a skateboard; three, his family would think I was crazy for doing such an outrageous hairdo on him and; and four, he was all talk. He would throw out crazy ideas, as if he were fishing and wanted to see if I would take the bait. I had news for him. Not only was I not taking the bait but I wasn't even on the same lake he was. He was on his own, and I learned to just override his ideas, knowing he just wanted a reaction from me.

He was talking as if he was serious about the Mohawk. He wanted to just see what it would look like, to shock his family, and he thought it would be funny to walk in the door at home and greet his wife. He asked if he got one, could he come back in tomorrow to have me cut the rest off, so he would just have a short hairdo all over. I went to my schedule to see if I had a time slot for such a service. I put him in at eleven o'clock in the morning. I proceeded to cut the Mohawk and, as I was making it stand on end, I remembered I had a couple of different hair mascaras. One was red, the other, gold. I talked him into letting me finish it with the color. I mean, if you were going to sport a Mohawk, you had to adorn it with some color. As he walked out, other stylists came back to the cutting area to see who had just cut that style. I was embarrassed to say, but owned up to it, letting them know it was what he truly wanted.

The next morning, as I pulled into work at nine thirty in the morning, I saw him sitting in the parking lot in his truck. He was wearing one of those hunter's hats with the long ear flaps. I told him he was early, that his appointment was not until eleven o'clock in the morning.

He said, "I need this thing off. I can wait." It was funny that he was not going to go anywhere until he got his hair fixed, even being at home was brutal, and I couldn't wait to hear more about it. He would rather sit in the parking lot, with a hot hat, on a summer's day, than be seen with this hairdo. When it was time for his appointment, I motioned for him to come in. I asked about the events of the Mohawk night. He told me he went to the grocery store after he left me, and as he was standing in line, an older man was staring at him.

He said to the older man, "What are you looking at?"

The man replied, "Aren't you a little old to be wearing spikes?"

He snapped back, "You have spikes coming out your nose!" I guessed the hairdo suited him. You have to have attitude to wear a Mohawk, and this client has major attitude. I used to call him the Barbarian. He would always speak his mind. I would constantly remind him it was time to change his filter, since words were slipping out, without any thought process. There was no holding back what was on his mind.

One day, as he was about to pay, he pulled out a one-hundred-dollar bill. I went to get change, but left the money with him. As I counted out the change, he took the change and the one-hundred-dollar bill.

I said, "Hey! Wait a minute! The one-hundred-dollar bill is mine. I am giving you change for it." I then counted it back to him, but he would not give me the one hundred dollars. I was getting a little testy with this game. It was not funny, and my next client was in. Did he think I had all day to play Who's on First with him, as if he were my only client?

I grabbed his hand, and with all my strength, pushing my thumb into his wrist, making him say, "Ouch!" I pushed even harder, until his hand opened up and the money fell onto my counter.

I grabbed it and told him, "Goodbye. Have a nice day." I'm always so darned polite.

I don't have time to play such games. Some days you have time to maybe look at your clients' pictures, or listen longer to their stories; other days you are on a tight schedule. I guess if you do it once, they are always going to think you have time the next time. Sometimes they know your next client is in, but they stay planted in your chair and don't want to leave. When I take the cape off, don't just sit there and cross your legs. Crossing your legs tells me you are getting comfortable, and when you are comfortable, you are not going to leave. Even though I have a schedule to keep, and may have another client waiting, I am happy they want to spend time with me, but come on. Your time is up. You are not the only one.

BREATH ALERT

We all know what it is like to feel trapped in a small space with bad breath. You just want to run, free yourself from the smell, and breathe again. When working with the public in close quarters, you need to be aware of your breath. You don't want to impose a bad breath encounter upon your client. I am good about not eating onions or garlic for lunch, and if I have it for dinner, I keep it in that day to fade away window. I don't want to offend my clients, so don't offend me. It is not good when you have to stand over someone and have to cut her bangs when she has "the breath." I have done it a few times where I have to say to myself, *"I'm going in…"* I take a deep breath and hold it, in hopes that I can cut the bang area before running out of air. It has to be the same for the client, if the stylist has bad breath, the clients are being held captive. What are they going to do? Leave in the middle of the cut? Say they forgot to turn off their iron? Besides, let's face it, who irons these days? Either way, it is not a pleasant experience.

I had a massage one day that was not a good experience, due to bad breath. She was considerably late starting with me, and it was my first time patronizing that spa. I sat in the waiting room for what felt like an eternity, trying to remain relaxed. When she finally got to me, she was frazzled and couldn't find the headrest part of the massage table. You need that part of the table so your head can stay aligned with your body. Why is it whenever there is an ad for a massage, the patron is lying with his or her head to the side and that part of the table is missing? So we can see the person's eyes are closed and he or she is smiling? Well the person won't be smiling after the massage when he or she has to get off the table after lying with his or her head cranked to the side. That person is going to need another massage.

I lay there, trying to be relaxed, waiting for her to come back into the room, ready for the pampering to begin. When she came back into the room and got ready to start, she sat behind my head as I lay on my back, and then the garlic punched me in the face. I wanted to plug my nose. Was this why she was late? Was she eating raw garlic with a side of sautéed onions? She kept telling me to relax and breathe in and out and then she started breathing in and out, spreading her garlic breath over me, as if it were a heavy blanket, the uncomfortable, scratchy kind that irritated your skin.

As I laid there, diminished of oxygen from holding my breath, I came close to telling her I could not breathe on account of the garlic cloud she cast out over me, ruining my Mother's Day pampering. It was a big, smelly elephant in the room. I could have almost seen it and would rather have had the smell of the elephant. Of course, I was supposed to relax, but I was thinking of an elephant and how it would make the room smell better. I thought it was just common sense to not have garlic for lunch when you are working with clients in close quarters.

Certain dinners would also linger and cause a garlic hangover. You couldn't be too careful. I worked with a stylist who had garlic hangovers all the time. Saturday mornings were the worst. I guessed the Friday night dining got a little carried away with the garlic. If people eat that much garlic, are they trying to ward off vampires? They are also warding off other humans and can only associate with their own kind. When two people eat garlic together, it cancels the garlic out, but then you cannot inflict this upon others who are not in your dining circle. It is best to wait it out, stay home, drink a lot of water, and get it out of your system before imposing your breath out in public.

The minute I would come into the salon on a Saturday morning and go around the corner to my station I would smell the garlic breath. I would make sure my clients knew it was not me. All of the stylists would gather in the break room and complain about it, open the doors, hoping to air it out a bit, and then we would wonder if it was time for an intervention, because mints couldn't cut this sharp odor that came out of nowhere and slapped you in the face. I would be mad all day, getting whiffs here and there. It could really make you bitter and angry. Bad odors, which are left to grate on your nerves for long periods of time, could make you feel this way.

I've been at the movie theater after just picking what I thought were fabulous seats when people came in after me and sat behind me, talking it up as if it were a continuation of dinner conversation, and then I smelled the garlic. Yes, they just came from dinner, and the mint that was offered to them did not do the trick. It seemed breath like that liked to move forward, not up. If it would just rise, I would be happy—since I'm shorter—but no, it seemed to have a purpose and move forward as if it was on a mission, projecting itself onward. *How long can I take this before I have to move?* I think. Not long.

Whenever any of us at work had an issue, we would say we were bitter and angry, taking it to that next level and making one another laugh. I would say it to some of my clients, and they thought it was funny. Something about saying you're bitter and angry makes you laugh, and you can no longer remain bitter or angry. Now when one of my clients told me a story that really got to her, she added she was bitter and angry. She had an unhappy marriage for as long as I could remember. She said she couldn't stand her husband or his behavior. She said she was going to write his obituary then, while she had a few nice things to say about him, because as the days went by, she was finding less good in him and would not have a single kind word to say about him when the time did come to write his obituary. I hope I don't get questioned from the police one day if he passes unexpectedly, since clients confess things to their hair stylists.

I was over at a client's house for dinner one evening, and as we were sitting around the table, enjoying our meal, I could smell the family dog at my feet. The dog was an old Saint Bernard. He had the hottest, smelliest breath, and I could not eat my dinner, because all I could smell was his breath. It felt hot against my legs. I could almost feel condensation forming to my lotion-covered legs, making them dewy. I knew he was under the table but didn't want to offend my client. I came up with a clever plan to get her to notice the dog was under the table, breathing on me and ruining my dining experience. I asked her if there was a heat vent under the table by my feet, that I was feeling some hot air. I got her to look under the table, and she saw the dog, hovering around my legs. As my plan unfolded, she removed the dog, making him go lay down in the other room, and I was rescued. Later I told her about the incident and that I knew he was there, that I didn't want to offend her, but I could not take another bite since his breath was so bad. She was not offended. She said that she knew how bad the dog's breath was and would make sure not to have him in the room if I ever came back for dinner. Interestingly, I was never invited back.

I had a new client in one day, and the minute I greeted him, I could smell his hot garlic breath. I tried to pretend it wasn't bothering me, but as time went on, I was close to telling him I could not finish his cut. While he lay back in the shampoo bowl, he talked, and the smell rose to my face, making it the fastest shampoo I've ever performed. I tried to be quiet, and not ask him about himself, to cut down on the amount of time his mouth would open. I have never, in all of my cutting years, smelled garlic breath that potent. The next time he was on my schedule, I was dreading his arrival, but luckily, the garlic was finally at bay.

THE ONE WHO GOT AWAY

It is a natural thing, yet we are so cautious not to share it with the world, but it slips out anyway. Sometimes, you can get lucky and it will go unnoticed, other times, not so lucky.

It happened to me one time. Only once, and it was not as though I meant for it to happen. We don't mean for these things to happen; they just do. I had one slip out. I prayed to the gas gods it would be OK, but then it hit. If I could smell it, I knew my client could smell it since she was sitting down lower than me. I was sure it hit her first, and yet she was so composed. I looked around quickly to see if I could blame it on someone doing a perm, since perms always had that lingering sulfur smell, but there was no one else in the room but my client and me. I was in the middle of telling her a story but lost my words and was unaware of what to do. My face was turning red, and I was stuttering. I wondered if I should just admit it and lead her out of the area until the coast was clear, have a little laugh, and feel I did the polite thing, but something inside me didn't want to own up to it. There was still a chance she was unsure of where it came from. We do that thing where we tell ourselves that if we don't acknowledge it, it wasn't ours, as if the other person is the only one with the smelling issue. I then lowered in the mirror, lining my face up with the back of her head, blocking my visibly red face and my guilty expression. I pretended to look at the neckline of her haircut, even though I had moved past that section long before. Thank goodness it dissipated, and things got back to normal.

Someone in the salon would be doing a perm, and the smell would drift over just enough to make you wonder if your client had gas. It then dawned on you that if you were thinking that, then the client was thinking it too. You would look around, find the culprit, and make sure the client knew the source of the foul smell.

I was talking to another stylist about these mishaps, and she said that she let them go all the time. If she was blow-drying, she guided the air into another direction. I used to work next to her. She did a lot of perms. I thought it was the perm I was smelling. Mystery solved. I actually thought it was her clients since they were older, and they would pass gas as they walked by my station. She said she also sprays hairspray to mask the smell if needed. It seemed she had it all worked out.

When I was in fourth grade, I was standing with my mom at the checkout counter of our grocery store. I let one go that was awful, I couldn't bear it myself to stay there. I told my mom I was going to wait in the car. I was relieved to get away from the odor, leaving the scene, as I waited in the car, singing, forgetting all about it.

The first thing my mom said to me was, "We knew it was you."

Those are haunting words. I thought I got away with it. I said, "It wasn't me."

My mom said, "We knew it was you because you left, and you know what I'm talking about."

There was nothing else I could say in my defense, and I learned a valuable lesson that day. As a grown-up, I would go places with my mother-in-law, and she would never hold back. We would be standing there when I would detect it the moment people approached us. I remembered what my mom had said, so I couldn't leave. I had to stand there in it because I was afraid of walking away and leaving them to think it was me.

Now, I work in a studio all by myself. I had a woman in my chair with the door closed when it hit me. There was no denying what happened: she passed gas. I didn't want to embarrass her, but I was hoping she would own up to it so I wouldn't have to stand in it, but she didn't. It wouldn't go away, so I was fighting for air for a good ten minutes. What if the tables were turned? The client would know it was from me since we were the only ones in the room. There were pros and cons to having my own space.

I had a boy in, the age of eight. I had him sit on a board that rests on the armrests of my chair so I could reach him better. One day, as he was sitting on the board, he was acting bored and leaning forward, tolerating his haircut. I was holding a conversation with his father, who was on the couch. The smell hit me like a smack in the face, causing me to jump back to address the horrific odor.

The boy said, "I held it as long as I could."

I told him, "Next time, just tell me. Think about it. Your bottom is higher than normal. You are leaning forward. The smell rose directly into my face."

I was out of the room so fast, trying to get some air as I exhaled long puffs out through my nose, trying to free the smell. I started to go back in, but there was no way, since it was still in there, as if it was trapped like a genie in a bottle. His dad was covering his face, laughing hysterically. When it was safe to go back in, I grabbed the air freshener. The boy then added, "They fed me chili." The next time he was in, I greeted him with a hair clip on my nose and told him I was ready to cut his hair.

I had another little boy in who was sitting on my couch awaiting his turn as I cut his father's hair. He was playing a video game on an iPad when I heard the noise against the leather. I looked at him. He acted as if it was no big deal, just a natural thing. I had to address it and say, "Are you breaking in my couch? I haven't even broken in my couch yet." His father told him to say, "Excuse me," and then we moved on.

Another man was in my studio, sitting on my couch. I had already cut his hair and was finishing up with his wife. He announced he had to go to the bathroom. He struggled to get up, reaching for his cane. His leg was a little wobbly, and his wife told him to get his balance before he took a step. I looked at him; his leg was shaking. I looked back at what I was doing when I heard him pass gas, followed by a "whoops." He then moved on out of the room, closing the door behind him. I went over to the door and said we could leave it open. I saw him walk toward the bathroom, and I said, "So we can get some fresh air." His wife and I started laughing. I guess people were comfortable with me, but I never want that comfort.

Another lady who was in was telling me a story, starting out with how it was a two-parter. The first part was that she had bad gas one night at home and her husband came home, walking in from the fresh air, and said, "What, are you crop dusting the whole downstairs?" Then the next night, still gassy and trying to be polite, she said she let it go in the vacuum hose. I took a moment to think about what she was saying, and of course, I pictured it.

She then said, with a smirk on her face, "It didn't work."

I said, "Was it a Dyson? Because if it was a Dyson, I bet it would work."

She said, "It was a Shark."

At this point, I was laughing so hard I could not continue my work.

It usually never happened to me, but it was just my luck that the one time it had to happen, there was no one else around, no perm to blame it on. I know it happens. Even the pope does it.

GONE BUT NOT FORGOTTEN

Well, my client passed away, and it turned out he did not have in his will that I would have to cut his hair one last time before he was buried. All of those years, I thought he was preparing me for the casket cut, reassuring me that I would be summoned to the task. I had to admit, I was very relieved.

He called me one Sunday night, telling me he had about a week to live. I was a little surprised and shocked by his news, but I had watched him decline the previous year, and it had left me curious. He had not been able to drive to his hair appointments, so I would go to his place to cut his hair. He told me he was at the VA Hospital, and I promised to visit him the next day. I hung up and just cried for him. My heart was truly breaking with the events unfolding before me. I had cut his hair for so long, but it went way beyond that. John was like family to me.

As I entered his room and he lay in bed, I reminded myself to stay strong and act as though nothing was wrong. I wanted our visit to be casual, as if we were just hanging out in a normal setting, but the thing was, I had never seen him lying in a hospital bed hooked up to IVs. We exchanged pleasantries, and I filled him in on the new things in my life. Then he got up so he could show me the view from the main window. It was pretty spectacular, and I wished I was enjoying it on different terms. As I said goodbye and left, I wondered if this would be the last time I saw him.

He then went home, and I made a plan to go visit and take him some homemade soup. As I walked into his home, I thought to myself that he looked good. Better than he did at the hospital. Abby was there from hospice care, and they were discussing cremation plans. While trying to tune the conversation out, I busied myself in the kitchen in search of a bowl to use to heat the soup I made. When it was warm, I handed it to him and sat down and joined the conversation that was going on. It was not a fun one. As I was getting ready to leave, I mentioned that he looked good, and that his hair was long. I asked him if he would be up to getting a haircut. It might have made him feel better.

He replied that he wasn't feeling up to it. Then continued, "You will get around to it." I knew what he was talking about; it was morbid, but it told me he was feeling better.

I said, "I will not cut your hair then. I just heard you were going to be cremated anyway."

He said, "I want to look good for when I'm cremated."

I added, "To the end. You are joking to the end." As I left, I actually felt it would be the last time I saw him. I was right.

When I walked into the church for his celebration-of-life service, I tried to remain strong. I looked at all the photos of him that were displayed for our viewing, but I felt out of place, only because I felt everyone was probably wondering who I was. I stood at the door to go in, waiting for the greeter to hand me one of the envelopes he was passing out, but for some reason, he wouldn't hand me one. He just seemed to stand there, looking at me, so I took it as my cue and went in to take a seat, trying not to draw any attention to myself. I noticed the other people seated in the rows ahead of me were looking at a photo of him from the envelope. I decide to go back to the main door greeter to get one. I took my seat again and opened the envelope, pulling out the picture. As I looked at it and read about his life, I couldn't control the force of tears that took over, holding my emotions hostage. I was in full cry stage. I saw his daughter enter the church, and she and her family were seated in the front.

Sitting there, listening to the service, another wave of emotion took me over, and now I had gone through three Kleenex tissues. I needed to get control of myself before I saw his daughter. I wanted to be strong for her. She got up to say a few words, and as she spoke her emotions, I saw others wipe at their tears. I just felt for her and knew she and her father loved each other so very much. I wanted to tell John about this event, as if he were still here to share things with. He had been gone for four months, but I felt he was still around, bringing us all together.

When I moved to the reception, it hit me again, and I was full-on crying. It was like the dam had burst, and there was nothing that could hold it back. I had to leave. I barely made it to my car and had to wait for my eyes to clear before I could drive. *What a mess I am*, I thought. I was a little embarrassed. The only person who knew me was his daughter. I wondered if everyone was wondering who the heck that blonde gal was, crying for John? And then I thought how John would think that was funny.

Little things remind me of him: being blamed for someone having gray hair or an accusation that used to make him say, "Excuse me!" I smile and remember how special it was to have him in my chair all of those years. The clients become friends, then family, and they never leave you.

I had another client who passed. She gave me a nice Santa candle for Christmas years ago. I get it out every year and put it in a sleigh with candy and think of her. Also, I cannot throw out their cards from my client card box. From time to time, I thumb through client cards and run across a client who is gone. I usually take a moment to think of him or her. I share stories with my clients about a client who has passed. It is my grieving process, I guess. My clients mean a lot to me.

Another older lady client of mine was dying. I would go to her house to visit, to take her a little sunshine. One Sunday afternoon, as she lay in her bed, she told me she had some champagne in her refrigerator, and she asked me if I wanted some. I really didn't, and it didn't register to me that she wanted to share some with me, so we didn't end up having any. I always felt bad about that.

After she passed, I went to take her husband some holiday goodies. I had been working so many hours, and I was exhausted and starving, wanting to get home to my family. He asked me to have some wine with him, and I remembered how I felt for passing before on the champagne with his wife, so I said I would have some with him. We made a toast, and as we were sitting there, he told me how he met Joyce and that he'd been married before. Then he said, "My first wife liked to have a lot of sex." Well, I didn't know quite what to say to that, so I just listened. When a seventy-nine-year-old man talks about his sex life, is it harmless? It went there again, and I was starting to feel uncomfortable.

He continued to tell me he worked in a library with a lot of women, and she was jealous, so she made sure he was satisfied before he left for work. I tried to change the subject and asked more about his marriage with Joyce. He told me their little story, and then said, "My first wife liked to have a lot of sex."

OK, now I was feeling that sufficient time had passed. I knew he was getting a little senile, so I chalked it up to that. I wished him a Merry Christmas, and was on my way. I had every intention of visiting him again, but when I called, the phone was disconnected. I never heard from him or knew who to call to find out, but I was always glad I had that time with him, for Joyce.

Another older lady client of mine Becky, passed just over a year ago, just two years after her husband, Pete. I used to go to their house to cut their hair. He was ninety-eight when he passed. He would take his hearing aids out, remove his glasses, and sit in the kitchen chair with two extra cushions, to be taller for me. Since he couldn't hear me, he would just sit there with his eyes closed, and he would have the biggest smile on his face. I would look at him and just say to myself, "Oh, look how cute he is, and how happy he is to be getting a haircut…Aww." I was usually there for quite a while, as they were slow moving.

One night I went over to their house with pizza for his ninety-second birthday. After we had dinner and were getting ready to cut the cake, I tried to help, but Becky would not have it. I wanted to be helpful so it would move along a little faster. I still had to cut their hair and had already worked a long day, and I was due back to work in the morning. Pete got up to scoop the ice cream, and as he did, he used a putty knife and scraped it out of the carton in long strips that were practically melting by the time he did four servings. When he finished, I peeked in the ice cream carton, and the remaining ice cream was flat, void of uneven scoop marks, appearing as a new carton. I had never seen anything like that, and I, myself, was type A. As we sat at the table, Becky started serving the cake, and after each slice, she licked her fingers. I tried not to let this bother me, but my daughter was also there, and I just knew she would not eat her cake after witnessing that serving style. She made a comment that she was full, so Becky ended up giving her a little doggy bag for her cake. After dinner and haircuts, my daughter and I were there four hours. It was a long night, but they were a sweet couple, and when I think of them, I have such love in my heart

Not long ago, another lady client passed away. She called to tell me she had a brain tumor and she was going to start chemotherapy and needed to cancel her hair appointment. I ended up shaving her head since her hair was falling out. She took a turn for the worse and was in hospice care. She was very dear to me, as she was a mother figure. She was always fun and would say exactly what was on her mind, and she was known for hitting people. I would say something like, "You have to uncross your legs now, since I am going to start cutting." She would give me a look, and I would say, "Just don't hit me." Then she would. One day, we were at the reception area, getting ready to say goodbye. We usually hugged, but she kissed me, right square on the mouth. I was shocked, and looked at the three other ladies who were standing behind the desk, their faces holding a little shock as well. She turned and left, and we all started laughing. I went to my station and saw she had left her water bottle behind, but I was afraid to call her, thinking she might kiss me again.

I called her, and she answered, "I left my water bottle, I know." She always left her water bottle.

I said, "I wasn't sure about calling you and having you come back, because I didn't want you to kiss me again."

She said, "Oh, shut up. You are like my daughter." So I always joked with her that she could hug me goodbye, just don't kiss me! Then I would move out of the way of her hitting hand. She had so much energy, whenever she left, I felt as if my batteries were recharged.

Ten days after she was in hospice care, it was her birthday. I knew she was comatose, but wanted to see her. We had snow on the ground, and the roads were still icy. It took me a while to get to her, and I ended up parking and walking the rest of the way, but I was able to make it in. When I first got there, her boyfriend said to her, "Debbie is here to do your hair." Since she was bald at that point, it made me laugh, because I knew she would find the humor in it. The next day, she passed, and I would forever be grateful I made it that day, that special birthday for Linda, to kiss her on the cheek and tell her I loved her.

I recently lost another close client. She had been in my chair for over nineteen years, and she came in every three weeks, so I knew her quite well. I am just at a loss and am reminded to let those people know I love them. I will remember all of the heart-to-heart talks we had and how we always solved our problems and the problems of others. She always wanted to help me with things and was such a fantastic gardener. She gave me starts from some of her outdoor plants, so now when I look at them, I will really cherish them. She came over one day to help me get rid of a mole. She was an expert at removing moles from the premises, and she didn't let me down. I have many memories of her, that I will hold onto. – for Patti

The thing is, the little reminders of them are nice, but I don't need reminders to remember them. They remain forever in my heart; they are part of memories that shape who I am as a person. They will always be with me.

I am so lucky, to have the job I love. My passion for hair has only gotten stronger over the years.

I am thankful for my trusting, loyal clients, and know I owe it all to you. I thank each one of you for your continued support, and for believing in me. My door is open — My shears are sharp –My heart is full.

ABOUT THE AUTHOR

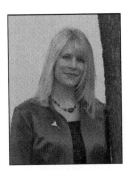 Debbie McRoberts has always been passion-
ate about hairstyling. She grew up in a small
town but moved to a large city to attend beauty
school.

McRoberts's new collection of anecdotes comes
from thirty-two years on the job. She believes
her job isn't just to ensure that her clients look
amazing but also to make them laugh.

Denice,
Thank you for
all of your support
+ love... and massages!
Happy reading!
love,
Debbie
McRoberts

Made in the USA
San Bernardino, CA
25 July 2017